# TELEMEDICINE
Opportunities and developments in Member States

Report on the second global survey on eHealth

Global Observatory for eHealth series - Volume 2

# Acknowledgments

This publication is part of a series of reports based on the second Global Observatory on eHealth (GOe) Survey. The preparation of this report would not have been possible without the input of hundreds of eHealth experts and the support of the numerous colleagues at the World Health Organization headquarters, regional, and country offices.

Our sincere gratitude goes to over 800 eHealth experts in 114 countries worldwide who helped shape this report by sharing their knowledge through completing the survey. We are also indebted to an extensive network of eHealth professionals and WHO staff who assisted with the design and implementation of the survey. Names of contributors can be found at http://www.who.int/goe.

Special thanks to the many authors and reviewers who contributed their time and ideas to this publication including: Kendall Ho, Jennifer Cordeiro, Ben Hoggan, Helen Novak Lauscher, Francisco Grajales, Lisa Oliveira, and Andrea Polonijo of the eHealth Strategy office, University of British Columbia, Canada. The text was reviewed by international telemedicine experts including Richard Wootton, Antoine Geissbuhler, and Najeeb Al-Shorbaji.

Design and layout of this publication were managed by Messagio Studios and Jillian Reichenbach Ott. Editing was completed by Kai Lashley. Their efforts are appreciated.

The global survey and this report were prepared and coordinated by the WHO Global Observatory for eHealth: Misha Kay, Jonathan Santos, and Marina Takane.

# Contents

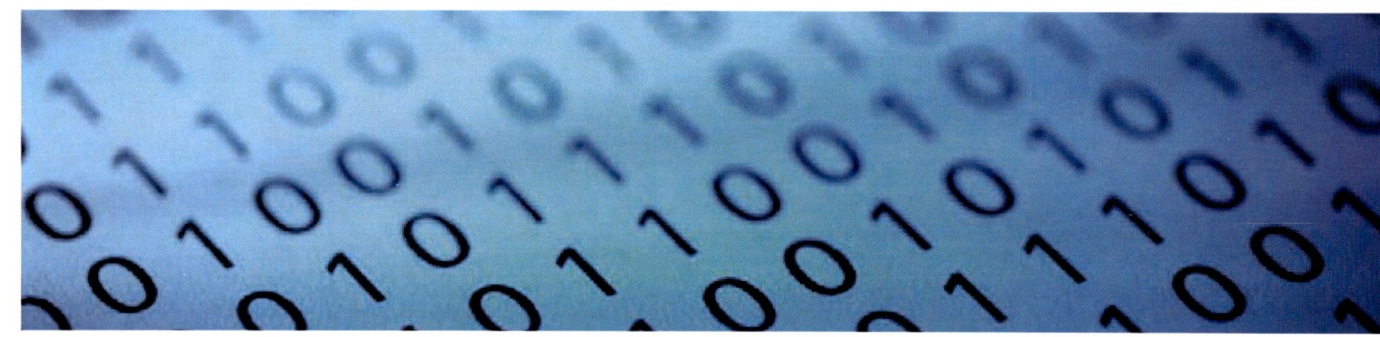

Acknowledgments .................................................................................................................. 3

Contents ................................................................................................................................... 4

Executive summary ................................................................................................................. 6

1. Introduction: Overview of telemedicine ........................................................................... 8
   1.1 What is telemedicine? ................................................................................................... 8
   1.2 Origins and history ........................................................................................................ 9
   1.3 Applications and services for diverse contexts ........................................................ 10
   1.4 Potential barriers to telemedicine diffusion ............................................................. 11

2. Telemedicine in developing countries: A review of the literature ............................... 12
   2.1 Literature review methodology .................................................................................. 12
      2.1.1 Study inclusion criteria ......................................................................................... 12
      2.1.2 Study exclusion criteria ........................................................................................ 13
      2.1.3 Literature search strategy .................................................................................... 13
      2.1.4 Selection of studies ............................................................................................... 13
   2.2 Telemedicine in developing countries: framing the survey findings .................... 13
      2.2.1 Opportunities for developing countries .............................................................. 13

Telemedicine supports maternal and newborn health in Mongolia ................................. 16
    2.2.2 Barriers to realizing the promise of telemedicine in developing countries ........... 18

Breast cancer screening for rural Mexican residents ........................................................ 20
    2.2.3 Legal and ethical considerations for telemedicine in developing countries ......... 22
    2.2.4 Implications for telemedicine development, implementation, evaluation, and sustainability ........................................................................................................................ 23
    2.2.5 Key lessons from the literature ................................................................................ 23

# 3. GOe Second Global Survey on eHealth .................................................................. 28

## 3.1 Survey implementation ........................................................................................ 29
    3.1.1 Survey instrument ................................................................................................... 29
    3.1.2 Survey development ............................................................................................... 30
    3.1.3 Data collector .......................................................................................................... 30
    3.1.4 Launching the 2009 survey .................................................................................... 31
    3.1.5 Limitations ............................................................................................................... 32
    3.1.6 Data processing ....................................................................................................... 33

# 4. Telemedicine results ..................................................................................................... 36

## 4.1 Current state of telemedicine services ................................................................ 36
    4.1.1 Telemedicine services globally ............................................................................... 37
    4.1.2 Telemedicine services by WHO region .................................................................. 38
    4.1.3 Telemedicine services by World Bank income group .......................................... 40
    4.1.4 Other telemedicine initiatives occurring around the world ............................... 43

Norway's teleECG initiative ........................................................................................ 46
    4.1.5 Implications for telemedicine services .................................................................. 49

## 4.2 Factors facilitating telemedicine development ................................................... 50
    4.2.1 Governance .............................................................................................................. 50
    4.2.2 Policy and strategy .................................................................................................. 52
    4.2.3 Scientific development ........................................................................................... 58
    4.2.4 Evaluation processes .............................................................................................. 60

The Swinfen Charitable Trust Telemedicine Network ............................................... 62

## 4.3 Barriers to telemedicine ....................................................................................... 66
    4.3.1 Implications for barriers to telemedicine .............................................................. 72

## 4.4 Telemedicine information needs ......................................................................... 73
    4.4.1 Implications for the information needs of telemedicine ..................................... 79

# 5. Discussion and recommendations ............................................................................ 80

## 5.1 The current state of telemedicine services .......................................................... 80
    5.1.1 Factors facilitating telemedicine development .................................................... 80
    5.1.2 Barriers to telemedicine development ................................................................. 82

# 6. References ..................................................................................................................... 84

# 7. Appendix 1 .................................................................................................................... 88

# Executive summary

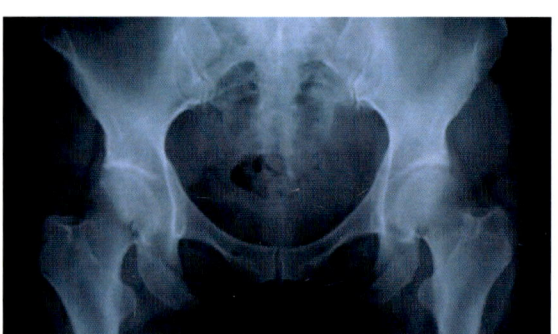 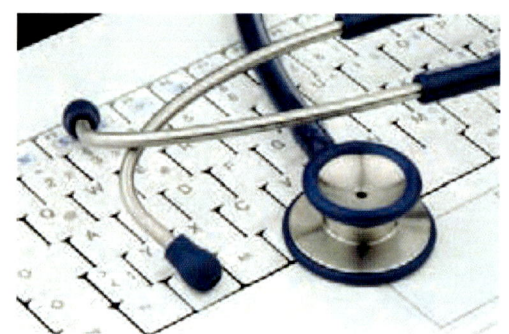 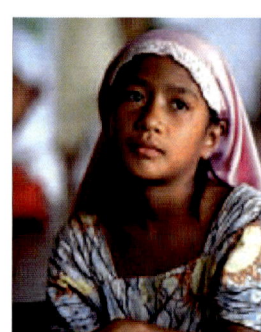

Information and communication technologies (ICTs) have great potential to address some of the challenges faced by both developed and developing countries in providing accessible, cost-effective, high-quality health care services. Telemedicine uses ICTs to overcome geographical barriers, and increase access to health care services. This is particularly beneficial for rural and underserved communities in developing countries – groups that traditionally suffer from lack of access to health care.

In light of this potential, the World Health Organization (WHO) established the Global Observatory for eHealth (GOe) to review the benefits that ICTs can bring to health care and patients' well-being. The Observatory is charged with determining the status of eHealth solutions, including telemedicine, at the national, regional, and global level, and providing WHO's Member States with reliable information and guidance on best practices, policies, and standards in eHealth.

In 2005, following the formation of WHO's eHealth strategy, the Observatory conducted a global eHealth survey to obtain general information about the state of eHealth among Member States. Based on the data from that survey, the GOe carried out a second global survey in 2009; it was designed to explore eight thematic areas in detail, the results of each being reported and analysed in individual publications – *the Global Observatory for eHealth series*.

The *eHealth series* is primarily meant for government ministries of health, information technology, and telecommunications, as well as others working in eHealth – academics, researchers, eHealth professionals, nongovernmental organizations, and donors.

The telemedicine module of the 2009 survey examined the current level of development of four fields of telemedicine: teleradiology, teledermatogy, telepathology, and telepsychology, as well as four mechanisms that facilitate the promotion and development of telemedicine solutions in the short- and long-term: the use of a national agency, national policy or strategy, scientific development, and evaluation. Telemedicine - opportunities and developments in Member States discusses the results of the telemedicine module, which was completed by 114 countries (59% of Member States).

Findings from the survey show that teleradiology currently has the highest rate of established service provision globally (33%). Approximately 30% of responding countries have a national agency for the promotion and development of telemedicine, and developing countries are as likely as developed countries to have such an agency. In many countries scientific institutions are involved with the development of telemedicine solutions in the absence of national telemedicine agencies or policies; while 50% of countries reported that scientific institutions are currently involved in the development of telemedicine solutions, 20% reported having an evaluation or review on the use of telemedicine in their country published since 2006.

The importance of evaluation within the field of telemedicine cannot be overstated: the field is in its infancy and while its promise is great, evaluation can ensure maximization of benefit. ICTs can be costly, as can be the programmes using them to improve health outcomes. Indeed, the most frequently cited barrier to the implementation of telemedicine solutions globally is the perception that the cost of telemedicine is too high.

Closely linked with cost is cost-effectiveness. Almost 70% of countries indicated the need for more information on the cost and cost-effectiveness of telemedicine solutions, and over 50% wanted more information on the infrastructure necessary to implement telemedicine solutions. Wanting additional information on the clinical uses of telemedicine was cited by almost 60% of countries; it was one of the three most requested areas of information by Member States.

While developing countries are more likely to consider resource issues such as high costs, underdeveloped infrastructure, and lack of technical expertise to be barriers to telemedicine, developed countries are more likely to consider legal issues surrounding patient privacy and confidentiality, competing health system priorities, and a perceived lack of demand to be barriers to telemedicine implementation.

Following the analysis of the survey results, WHO recommends steps Member States can take to capitalize on the potential of ICTs. One such step is creation of national agencies to coordinate telemedicine and eHealth initiatives, ensuring they are appropriate to local contexts, cost-effective, consistently evaluated, and adequately funded as part of integrated health service delivery. Ultimately telemedicine initiatives should strengthen – rather than compete with – other health services.

# 1 Introduction: Overview of telemedicine

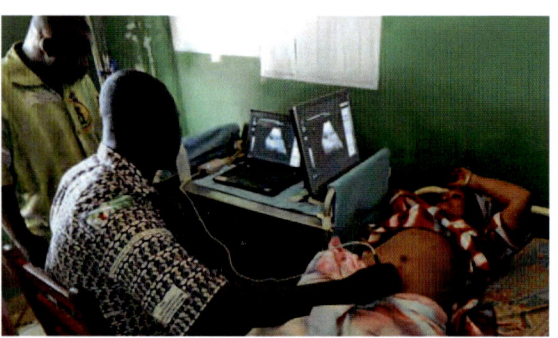 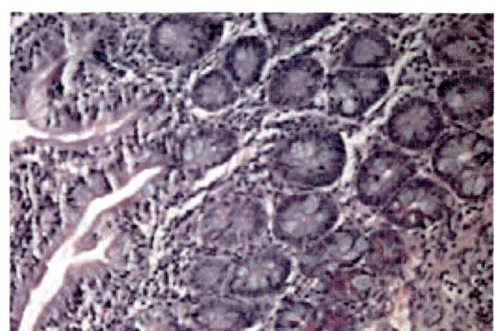 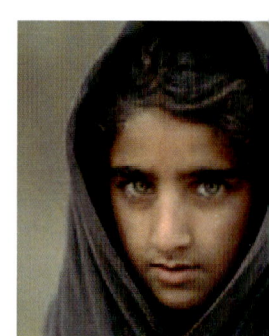

Access, equity, quality, and cost-effectiveness are key issues facing health care in both developed and less economically developed countries. Modern information and communication technologies (ICTs), such as computers, the Internet, and cell phones, are revolutionizing how individuals communicate with each other, seek and exchange information, and enriching their lives. These technologies have great potential to help address contemporary global health problems.

Rooted in the second global survey of eHealth conducted in 2009, this report focuses on the use of ICT for health service delivery—telemedicine. It begins by giving an overview of telemedicine, synthesizing current literature that illuminates the use of telemedicine in developing countries, and highlighting five key lessons learnt from this body of literature. The results of the Telemedicine Section of the second global eHealth survey are then discussed, and key findings highlighted. Finally, recommendations are made on the actions the World Health Organization and its Member States can take to establish telemedicine as part of a sustainable solution to the health care issues faced by developing countries. This unique examination, considering current ICT and the survey results, will provide innovative approaches to help conceptualize solutions to contemporary global health issues.

## 1.1 What is telemedicine?

Telemedicine, a term coined in the 1970s, which literally means "healing at a distance" (1), signifies the use of ICT to improve patient outcomes by increasing access to care and medical information. Recognizing that there is no one definitive definition of *telemedicine* – a 2007 study found 104 peer-reviewed definitions of the word (2) – the World Health Organization has adopted the following broad description:

*"The delivery of health care services, where distance is a critical factor, by all health care professionals using information and communication technologies for the exchange of valid information for diagnosis, treatment and prevention of disease and injuries, research and evaluation, and for the continuing education of health care providers, all in the interests of advancing the health of individuals and their communities" (3).*

The many definitions highlight that telemedicine is an open and constantly evolving science, as it incorporates new advancements in technology and responds and adapts to the changing health needs and contexts of societies.

Some distinguish telemedicine from telehealth with the former restricted to service delivery by physicians only, and the latter signifying services provided by health professionals in general, including nurses, pharmacists, and others. However, for the purpose of this report, telemedicine and telehealth are synonymous and used interchangeably.

Four elements are germane to telemedicine:

1. Its purpose is to provide clinical support.
2. It is intended to overcome geographical barriers, connecting users who are not in the same physical location.
3. It involves the use of various types of ICT.
4. Its goal is to improve health outcomes.

## 1.2 Origins and history

Historically, telemedicine can be traced back to the mid to late 19th century (4) with one of the first published accounts occurring in the early 20th century when electrocardiograph data were transmitted over telephone wires (5). Telemedicine, in its modern form, started in the 1960s in large part driven by the military and space technology sectors, as well as a few individuals using readily available commercial equipment (4, 6). Examples of early technological milestones in telemedicine include the use of television to facilitate consultations between specialists at a psychiatric institute and general practitioners at a state mental hospital (7), and the provision of expert medical advice from a major teaching hospital to an airport medical centre (8).

Recent advancements in, and increasing availability and utilization of, ICTs by the general population have been the biggest drivers of telemedicine over the past decade, rapidly creating new possibilities for health care service and delivery. This has been true for developing countries and underserved areas of industrialized nations (9). The replacement of analogue forms of communication with digital methods, combined with a rapid drop in the cost of ICTs, have sparked wide interest in the application of telemedicine among health-care providers, and have enabled health care organizations to envision and implement new and more efficient ways of providing care (4, 6). The introduction and popularization of the Internet has further accelerated the pace of ICT advancements, thereby expanding the scope of telemedicine to encompass Web-based applications (e.g. e-mail, teleconsultations and conferences via the Internet) and multimedia approaches (e.g. digital imagery and video). These advancements have led to the creation of a rich tapestry of telemedicine applications that the world is coming to use.

## 1.3 Applications and services for diverse contexts

Telemedicine applications can be classified into two basic types, according to the timing of the information transmitted and the interaction between the individuals involved—be it health professional-to-health professional or health professional-to-patient (4). Store-and-forward, or asynchronous, telemedicine involves the exchange of pre-recorded data between two or more individuals at different times. For example, the patient or referring health professional sends an e-mail description of a medical case to an expert who later sends back an opinion regarding diagnosis and optimal management (10). In contrast, real time, or synchronous, telemedicine requires the involved individuals to be simultaneously present for immediate exchange of information, as in the case of videoconferencing (10). In both synchronous and asynchronous telemedicine, relevant information may be transmitted in a variety of media, such as text, audio, video, or still images. These two basic approaches to telemedicine are applied to a wide array of services in diverse settings, including teledermatology, telepathology, and teleradiology (6, 11).

The majority of telemedicine services, most of which focus on diagnosis and clinical management, are routinely offered in industrialized regions including, but not limited to the United Kingdom of Great Britain and Northern Ireland, Scandinavia, North America, and Australia (4, 12). In addition, biometric measuring devices such as equipment monitoring heart rate, blood pressure and blood glucose levels are increasingly used to remotely monitor and manage patients with acute and chronic illnesses. Some predict that telemedicine will profoundly transform the delivery of health services in the industrialized world by migrating health care delivery away from hospitals and clinics into homes (13).

In low-income countries and in regions with limited infrastructure, telemedicine applications are primarily used to link health-care providers with specialists, referral hospitals, and tertiary care centres (13). Even though low-cost telemedicine applications have proven to be feasible, clinically useful, sustainable, and scalable in such settings and underserved communities, these applications are not being adopted on a significant scale due to a variety of barriers (14).

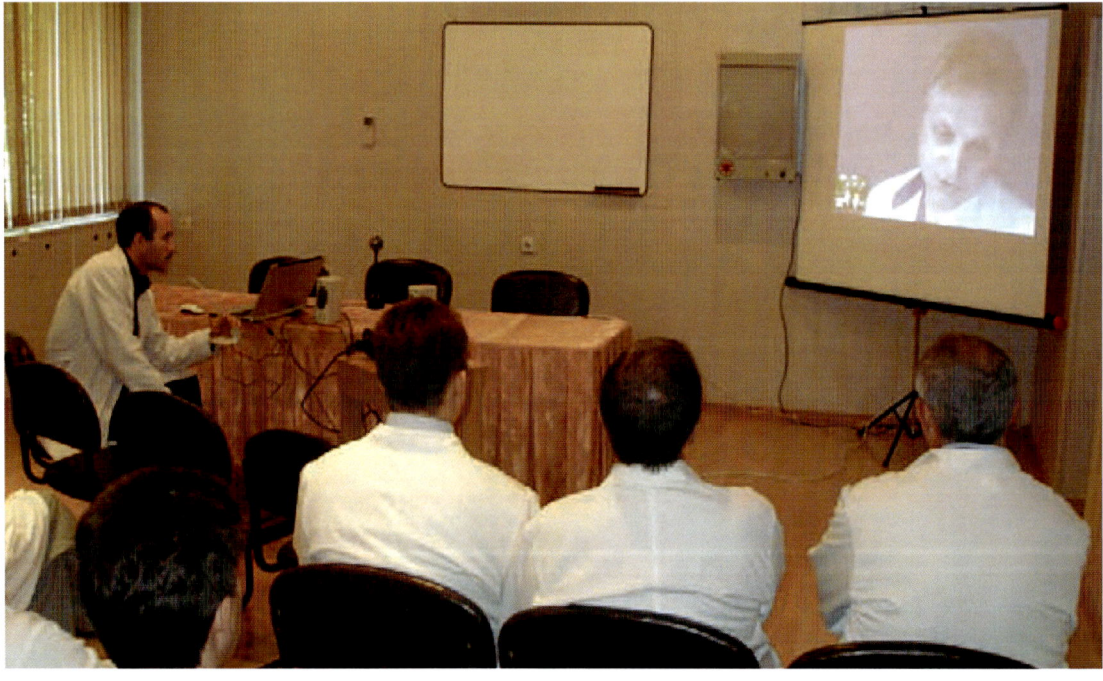

*Low-cost videoconferences are a powerful tool for clinical and learning objectives.*
*Photograph courtesy of Professor A. Vladzymyrskyy, Association for Ukrainian Telemedicine and eHealth Development, www.telemed.org.ua.*

## 1.4 Potential barriers to telemedicine diffusion

Telemedicine holds great potential for reducing the variability of diagnoses as well as improving clinical management and delivery of health care services worldwide by enhancing access, quality, efficiency, and cost-effectiveness (4, 13). In particular, telemedicine can aid communities traditionally underserved – those in remote or rural areas with few health services and staff – because it overcomes distance and time barriers between health-care providers and patients (4). Further, evidence points to important socioeconomic benefits to patients, families, health practitioners and the health system, including enhanced patient-provider communication and educational opportunities (15).

Despite its promise, telemedicine applications have achieved varying levels of success. In both industrialized and developing countries, telemedicine has yet to be consistently employed in the health care system to deliver routine services, and few pilot projects have been able to sustain themselves once initial seed funding has ended (14). Several routinely cited challenges account for the lack of longevity in many telemedicine endeavours.

One such challenge is a complex of human and cultural factors. Some patients and health careworkers resist adopting service models that differ from traditional approaches or indigenous practices, while others lack ICT literacy to use telemedicine approaches effectively. Most challenging of all are linguistic and cultural differences between patients (particularly those underserved) and service providers (4, 6, 13).

A shortage of studies documenting economic benefits and cost-effectiveness of telemedicine applications is also a challenge. Demonstrating solid business cases to convince policy-makers to embrace and invest in telemedicine has contributed to shortcomings in infrastructure and underfunding of programmes (4).

Legal considerations are a major obstacle to telemedicine uptake. These include an absence of an international legal framework to allow health professionals to deliver services in different jurisdictions and countries; a lack of policies that govern patient privacy and confidentiality vis-à-vis data transfer, storage, and sharing between health professionals and jurisdictions (16–18); health professional authentication, in particular in e-mail applications (17, 19); and the risk of medical liability for the health professionals offering telemedicine services (20).

Related to legal considerations are technological challenges. The systems being used are complex, and there is the potential for malfunction, which could trigger software or hardware failure. This could increase the morbidity or mortality of patients and the liability of health-care providers as well (20).

In order to over come these challenges telemedicine must be regulated by definitive and comprehensive guidelines, which are applied widely, ideally worldwide (21). Concurrently, legislation governing confidentiality, privacy, access, and liability needs to be instituted (22). As public and private sectors engage in closer collaboration and become increasingly interdependent in eHealth applications, care must be taken to ensure that telemedicine will be deployed intelligently to maximize health services and optimal quality and guarantee that for-profit endeavours do not deprive citizens access to fundamental public health services (22).

In all countries, issues pertaining to confidentiality, dignity, and privacy are of ethical concern with respect to the use of ICTs in telemedicine. It is imperative that telemedicine be implemented equitably and to the highest ethical standards, to maintain the dignity of all individuals and ensure that differences in education, language, geographic location, physical and mental ability, age, and sex will not lead to marginalization of care (22).

# 2 Telemedicine in developing countries: A review of the literature

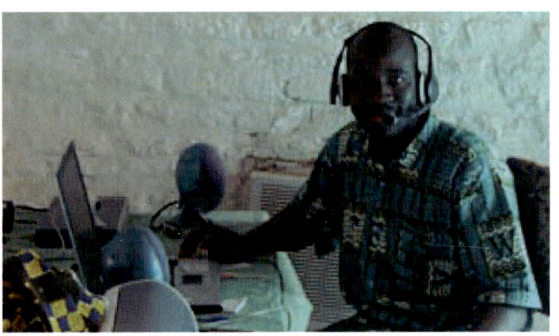
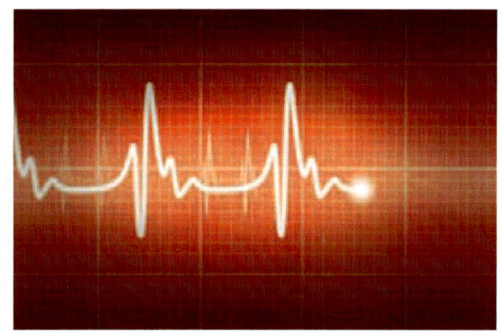
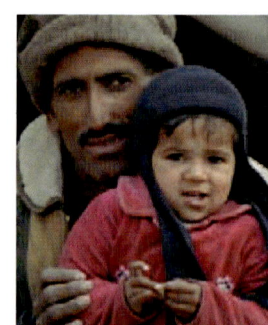

A systematic review of the literature was conducted to illuminate the current state of telemedicine in developing countries. Identified for review were studies that reported on patient outcomes, research and evaluation processes, education outcomes, and economic assessments.

## 2.1 Literature review methodology

### 2.1.1 Study inclusion criteria

Clinical studies, feasibility studies, and review articles were considered for inclusion, based on the criteria outlined below.

- Participants: the review included health-care practitioners from any medical discipline using telemedicine to treat patients in developing countries, and patients in developing countries receiving care through telemedicine, regardless of the origin of the service.
- Interventions: the review included studies examining any form of telemedicine application developed for, or involving developing countries.
- Outcomes: studies were included if they examined patient outcomes (including access to health care services and quality of health care), research and evaluation processes, or the education of health-care providers.
- Publication date: literature considered eligible for inclusion and critical appraisal was restricted to studies published from January 1999 onwards.
- Language: studies included were restricted to those published in English.

## 2.1.2 Study exclusion criteria

The review excluded studies which examined technical specifications (e.g. broadband requirements) of information and communications technologies used in telemedicine, and studies in which the primary purpose of telecommunications technology use was for administration, or was not linked to education or patient outcomes. The review also excluded studies that focused on mobile phones, personal digital assistants, remote patient monitoring devices, and other wireless devices to avoid duplication with the GOe report on mHealth to be published as a part of this eHealth series.

## 2.1.3 Literature search strategy

The Cochrane Database of Systematic Reviews, Medical Literature Analysis and Retrieval System Online (MEDLINE), Excerpta Medica Database (EMBASE), and Cumulative Index to Nursing and Allied Health Literature (CINAHL) databases were searched from January 1999 to January 2010 using the following search terms: 'telemedicine', 'developing countries' (medical subject heading terms); and 'telemedicine', 'tele*medicine', 'telehealth', 'tele*health', 'developing countr*', 'developing world' (text words).

The literature search further included searching of WHO regional indexes including African Index Medicus (AIM); the Eastern Mediterranean Region Library Network (EMLIBNET); Latin American and Caribbean Health Sciences (LILACS) produced by the Pan American Health Organization (PAHO) Institutional Memory Database; the WHO Library Database (WHOLIS); and the Western Pacific Region Index Medicus (WPRIM) using the WHO Global Health Library platform (www.globalhealthlibrary.net), and hand-searching of the telemedicine journals *Journal of Telemedicine and Telecare* and *Telemedicine Journal and e-Health* using terms corresponding to those listed above. It also included a limited search of references from retrieved articles. However, it did not include extended searching of Internet web sites and conference abstracts or contacting authors for unpublished data. Duplicate articles were excluded.

## 2.1.4 Selection of studies

Retrieved full-text studies were appraised to identify those to be included in the review. Full publications subsequently found not to meet the inclusion criteria were excluded.

Review results included 108 articles. Based on the criteria detailed above 27 of these were found not relevant and thus excluded from the review. The final number of articles included was 81.

## 2.2 Telemedicine in developing countries: framing the survey findings

### 2.2.1 Opportunities for developing countries

The literature reports that while telemedicine offers great opportunities in general, it could be even more beneficial for underserved and developing countries where access to basic care is of primary concern. One of the biggest opportunities telemedicine presents is increased access to health care. Providing populations in these underserved countries with the means to access health care has the potential to help meet previously unmet needs (23) and positively impact health services (24).

Telemedicine applications have successfully improved the quality and accessibility of medical care by allowing distant providers to evaluate, diagnose, treat, and provide follow-up care to patients in less-economically developed countries (*17, 25, 26*). They can provide efficient means for accessing tertiary care advice in underserved areas (*27*). By increasing the accessibility of medical care telemedicine can enable patients to seek treatment earlier and adhere better to their prescribed treatments (*28*), and improve the quality of life for patients with chronic conditions (*29*).

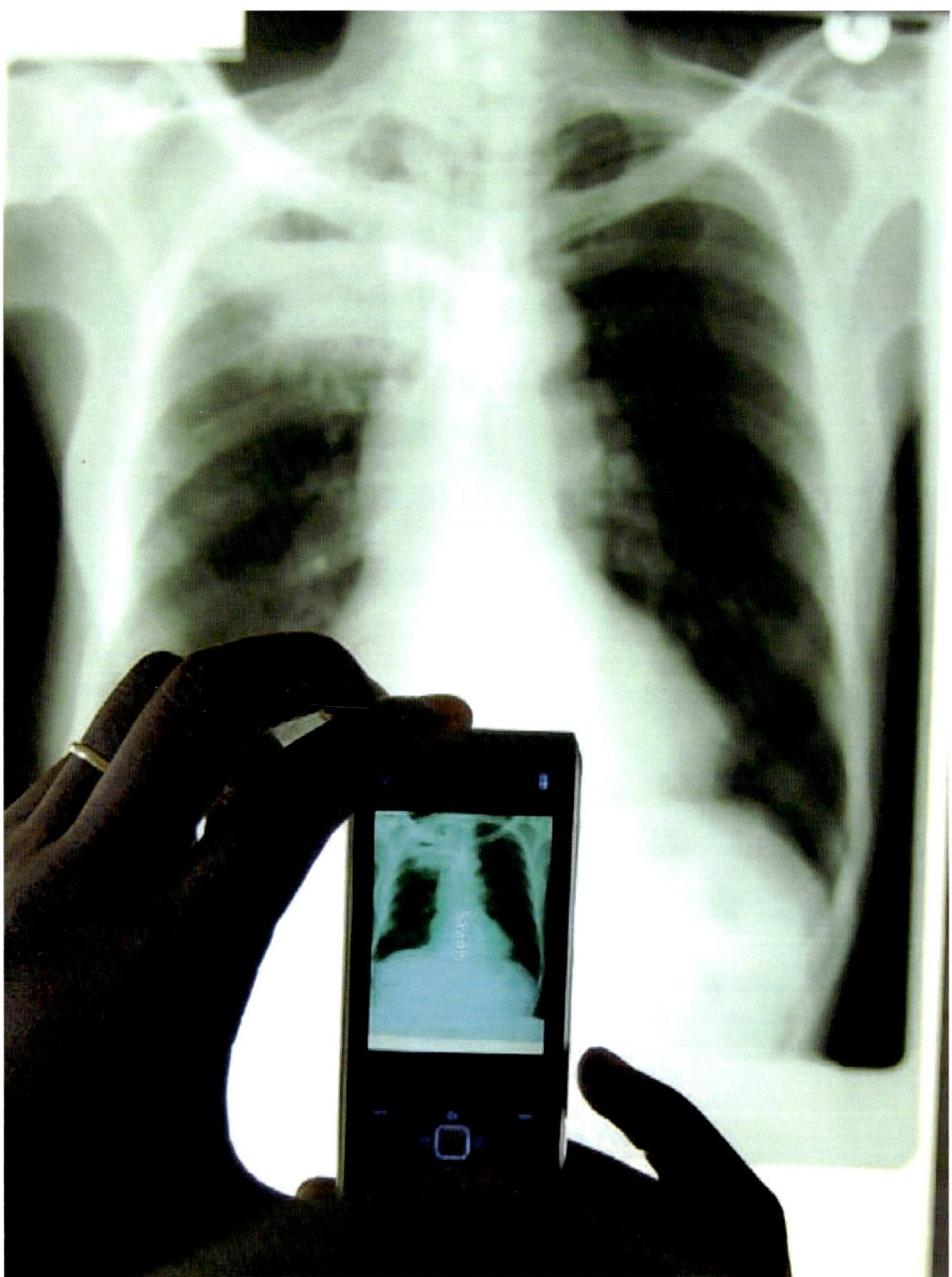

*Mobile teleradiology is utilized in villages in Botswana to communicate with radiologists in the capital city of Gaborone. (Photograph: Ryan Littman-Quinn, Carrie Kovarik: Botswana-UPenn Partnership)*

Telemedicine has been advocated in situations where the health professional on duty has little or no access to expert help (*30*); it is able to offer remote physician access to otherwise unavailable specialist opinions (*31*), providing reassurance to both doctors and patients. Telemedicine programmes have been shown to directly and indirectly decrease the number of referrals to off-site facilities and reduce the need for patient transfers (*32, 33*). Remote care and diagnosis via telemedicine in less-economically developed countries thus benefits both patients and the health care system by reducing the distance travelled for specialist care and the related expenses, time, and stress (*17, 29, 34, 35*). Furthermore, telemedicine programmes have the potential to motivate rural practitioners to remain in rural practice through augmentation of professional support and opportunities for continuing professional development (*36*).

Telemedicine networks in developing countries could also offer secondary benefits. Telecommunication technologies, such as those used in telemedicine initiatives, have shown to be effective tools for connecting remote sites (*37*). By opening up new channels for communication telemedicine connects rural and remote sites with health-care professionals around the world, overcoming geographical barriers and attempting to reverse 'brain drain' or flight of human capital (*25, 28, 34*). This can lead to increased communication between health service facilities, and facilitate cross-site and inter-country collaboration and networking (*17, 38*). Such collaborations can support health-care providers in remote locations through distance learning and training (*17, 31, 34, 39, 40*).

Telemedicine also provides opportunities for learning and professional development by enabling the provision and dissemination of general information and the remote training of health-care professionals (*41*). As Zbar and colleagues (*40*) asserted, "Telemedicine creates a university without borders that fosters academic growth and independence because the local participating surgeons have direct access to experts in the developed world." For example referred specialists have reported value in terms of medical education through the provision of consultation (*19*). It is important to note that such partnerships provide mutual benefits. For example, health-care providers in developed nations are provided with an opportunity to learn to treat neglected diseases, which they very seldom see in person (*38, 42, 43*).

The knowledge sharing that occurs as a result of inter-site collaboration may be formal or informal and has shown to aid health-care professionals in overcoming the professional isolation that they often face in remote areas, and to improve their skills and the services they offer (*44*). A telemedicine programme to support maternal and neonatal health in Mongolia (Case study 1) exemplifies many of these points.

# Telemedicine supports maternal and newborn health in Mongolia

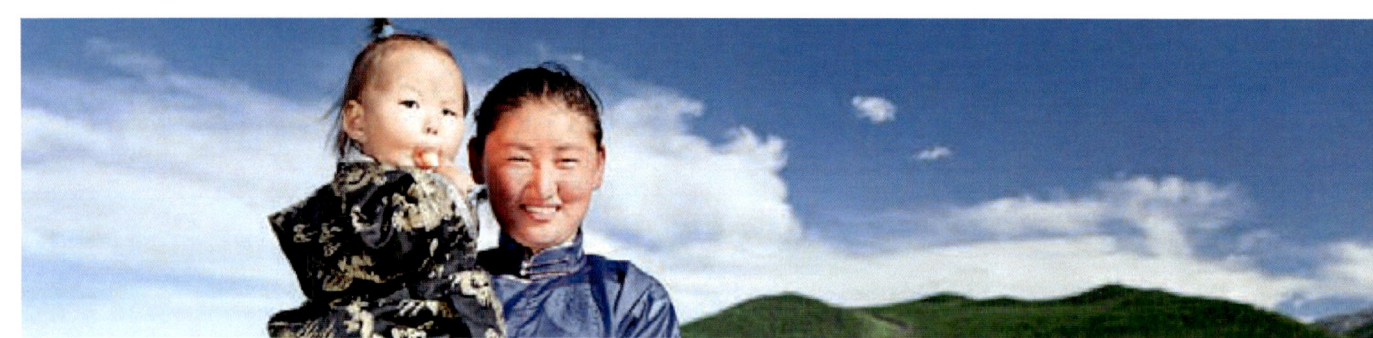

The aim of the Telemedicine Support to Promote Maternal and Newborn Health in Remote Provinces of Mongolia project is to reduce infant and maternal mortality while addressing the gap between urban and rural health care services. The project started in September 2007, and will continue to December 2010. The project's telemedicine services supports Aimags (provinces) with high-risk pregnancy consultations, prenatal ultrasound diagnostics, fetal monitoring, and screening for cervical abnormalities using colposcopy. The services provided by the project are particularly important for women in remote rural regions who do not have the funding to travel for expert opinion.

*There have been only two maternal deaths in the eight hospitals [involved in the programme]. Early diagnosis of fetal abnormalities is [now] possible in rural hospitals."*

—Dr Tsedmaa Bataar

A total of 297 doctors, nurses, and midwives were trained for this programme between March and December 2009. A total of 598 cases were referred in 2009. Of these, 64% were obstetrical, 21% were gynaecological pathology, and 15% were neonatal pathology. Only 36 of these cases were referred to Ulaanbaatar for treatment following the diagnosis, substantially saving the resources of rural residents that would otherwise have gone towards travel expenses.

*"Telemedicine support contributes to protecting people in rural areas from financial risks associated with travelling to Ulaanbaatar to obtain tertiary level maternal and newborn care."*

—Midterm Review Report Summary, June 2009

The success of this project is attributed to the hands-on training service model, a respect for local practices, and the knowledge base of local doctors. The project has fostered collaboration and an environment of mutual learning among health-care workers, and lessened the hierarchy often perceived between rural health-care staff and urban specialists, which has subsequently decreased the sense of isolation typically experienced by doctors working in rural areas.

The programme is not without its challenges. Barriers included equipment breakdowns (early use of inexpensive but low-quality goods may have compounded this problem); a lack of maintenance support in rural hospitals, IT specialists, and medical engineers; slow Internet bandwidth (sometimes too slow for synchronous connection); and some staff reported they were reluctant to change practice patterns and uptake new technologies.

Project funding was obtained through a joint venture among three agencies: the Mongolian Government's Mother and Child Health Research Centre (MCHRC) in Ulaanbaatar, the Government of Luxembourg (Lux-Development Agency), and the United Nations Population Fund (UNFPA). Regional hospitals in eight of the twenty-one Aimags are connected to the MCHRC through this project, and each regional hospital has two OBGYN project coordinators.

Due to the success of the programme, the UNFPA has extended project funding to Dec 2010 during which time an additional four regional hospitals from very remote Aimags will be included. With the aim to expand the project to include twelve of the twenty-one Aimags in Mongolia, the Mongolian Government has submitted a proposal to the Luxembourg Government for extended funding.

Acknowledgements
Dr Tsedmaa Bataar

Telemedicine can also support doctor-patient encounters in the long-term, as it provides health-care professionals with opportunities for case-based learning that can be applied in the treatment of future patients (45, 46). The introduction of technological resources that would be otherwise unavailable in the developing world additionally offers health-care professionals the opportunity to develop technological skills that are transferrable to other contexts (31).

Additionally, connecting multiple remote sites via telemedicine may prove to be a cost-effective way of delivering health care to these communities, when compared with the alternative of constructing facilities and hiring clinicians (47). Furthermore, such systems have great potential and applicability in the context of disasters where telecommunications can provide links between expert trauma centres and colleagues at the site.

Another tangential opportunity telemedicine offers developing countries is the ability to organize and collect patient data. Telemedicine tools and technology can help epidemiological surveillance by assisting in identifying and tracking public health issues and illustrating trends (39). Having the means to track this information allows for the monitoring of disease evolution and can support communication to plan and mobilize vaccination teams (24). Additionally, some systems can improve data management through network databases and electronic record keeping. This can help provide more coordinated care while also facilitating the potential for more patient follow-up and evaluation.

With progress in technology, the expansion of telemedicine in developing countries is promising, an example being the falling costs of ICTs (34, 41, 48–50). Others include increasing computing speeds, and options for high-speed bandwidth, and the falling costs of digital storage (51). Already, basic store-and-forward e-mail-based telemedicine requires minimal investment in hardware and software where network connectivity is available, and allows for detailed exchanges by enabling the transfer of images as attachments, making it an effective solution for low-resource settings (11, 17, 20, 52). The growing development of Internet-based conferencing (particularly through no-cost software) increases the accessibility and portability of conferencing and counters the need for expensive video conferencing equipment that may be limited in availability (53). Low bandwidth, Internet-based telemedicine (e.g., store and forward, e-mail-based consultations) has also proven to be a cost-effective technology that can efficiently and effectively pre-screen patients living in remote areas (54). By enhancing the information communication technology infrastructure and developing better communication facilities, telemedicine can also add to the better management of scarce medical resources and day-to-day activities in the developing world (17, 25).

### 2.2.2 Barriers to realizing the promise of telemedicine in developing countries

Infrastructure in developing countries is largely insufficient to utilize the most current Internet technologies. This lack, and inadequate access to computing are barriers to telemedicine uptake for many developing countries (24, 39, 51). At the most fundamental level, the instability of electric power supplies (18, 38, 55), widespread unavailability of Internet connectivity beyond large cities (38), and information and communication equipment that is not suitable for tropical climates (56) impose limitations on where telemedicine can be implemented. Unreliable connectivity, computer viruses, and limited bandwidth continue to present challenges when and where Internet access is available (19, 38, 53, 57, 58): Internet congestion can lead to delayed imaging (59); poor image resolution may limit the efficacy of remote diagnosis (60); and slow bandwidth can prohibit the use of real-time videoconferencing (61). Even when basic infrastructure is in place, widespread interoperability standards for software are lacking (57) and equipment or computer system failure remains an ever-present possibility (*17, 19*). Case study 2 highlights a programme in Mexico that has dealt successfully with the challenge of low bandwidth to provide breast cancer screening to rural residents.

Financial cost also poses both a real and perceived barrier to the application and adoption of telemedicine in developing countries (*55, 62, 63*). Equipment, transport, maintenance, and training costs of local staff can be daunting for countries with little income or limited funding for the implementation and maintenance of telemedicine initiatives (*16, 35, 39, 51, 59*). Moreover, convincing evidence to support the overall cost-effectiveness of particular telemedicine strategies may be weak (*64*), while the economic implications of such strategies in different settings may not yet be known (*18*).

Local skills, knowledge, and resources may also limit the application of telemedicine in developing countries. A lack of computer literate workers with expertise in managing computer services, combined with the lengthy process required to master computer-based peripheral medical instruments can hinder uptake (*63, 65*). While there may be a demand for distance learning, meeting local educational needs can be difficult due to differences in the diagnostic and therapeutic resources available, as well as the literacy and language skills across multiple sites (*51, 53, 55*). Moreover, while telemedicine may enhance expert diagnosis, treatment options available are constrained by logistical challenges including the training of local medical personnel, availability of medical equipment and supplies, and getting medicines to patients (*28, 66*).

Another barrier encountered is the sociocultural differences between sites, which can limit the pertinence of telemedicine collaborations in the developing world and challenge cultural perspectives related to health and wellness (*38, 51*). A major contributing factor to telemedicine failure is the oversight of incompatible cultural subsystems that prevent the transfer of knowledge from one cultural context to another (*2*). Medical professionals in the industrialized world may be unfamiliar with the available facilities and alternative management strategies in remote areas and vice versa (*60*). Telemedicine therefore risks the exchange of inappropriate or inadequate medical information (*38*). Without a good understanding of the local context, it may be difficult to integrate telemedicine in a useful way.

# Breast cancer screening for rural Mexican residents

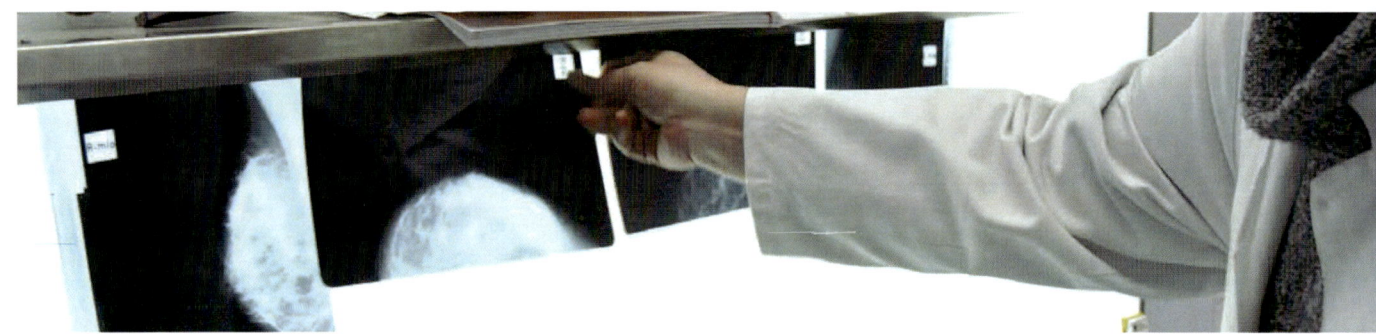

In 2006 breast cancer became the leading cause of death in Mexican women between the ages of fifty to sixty-nine. The Opportune Breast Cancer Screening and Diagnosis Program (OBCSDP) is meant to transcend economic and personnel barriers through the innovative deployment of ICTs. Aimed to reduce the breast cancer mortality rate in women between the ages of fifty to sixty-nine, the programme will increase the national screening rates from 7.2% in 2007 to 21.6% by 2012.

The telemedicine network had the goal to screen 1.3 million women in the 30-month period between May 2010 and December 2012. With over 34 million Mexican pesos (approximately US$ 2.8 million) of seed funding from the federal and state governments and not-for-profit groups, 30 screening sites in 11 states were linked by Internet to two interpretation centres, where results of the screenings could be viewed by radiologists. (In 2012, eight more interpretation sites will be opened, and the programme's operational costs will become self-sustaining.)

Due to challenges with Internet connectivity in rural areas of Mexico, many Mexican communities lack the necessary bandwidth for Internet protocol-based image transmission (necessary to transmit mammograms). To overcome this challenge, CDs were used for patient data transfer and long-term data (backup) storage. Each carried four patient images (a full mammography) and up to four patient mammograms. CDs are privately or commercially couriered to the closest interpretation centre (Phase 1). Results with this method, however, took up to three weeks to return to individuals.

Communities with Internet access will be evaluating individual partnership agreements with TelMex (a private telecom company) one calendar year after Phase 1 is initiated. If feasible, these should allow for instant data transfer between the screening and interpretation sites and will cut by half the picture-to-result time of 7–21 days required with the use of the CDs.

Quality control of hardware and its interoperability was also a challenge, as was standardizing the skill levels of radiology technicians. Scale up of the programme across Mexico was also a problem initially. The decentralization of partner institutions was also less than ideal, due to independent organizational structures, jurisdictional logistics, and funding schemes – all of which required extensive coordination and time to successfully overcome.

Two Secretary of Health subsidiary offices coordinated OBCSDP planning and coordination: the National Centre for Technological Excellence in Health (CENETEC), and the National Directorate for Gender Equity. These offices, along with several other groups facilitated this initiative financially and with other services.

This collaboration led to the programme overcoming a shortage of radiologists to improve equity of access in preventative breast cancer screening and diagnosis for rural and remote residents in over five states in Mexico.

Acknowledgements
Adrian Pacheco
Director, CENETEC

The adoption of telemedicine systems requires acceptance by both the patient and the health professional involved; both parties may be more familiar with face-to-face encounters and resistant to utilize telemedicine services, or unaware of their potential benefits (16, 51, 63, 67, 68). In particular, health-care professionals have reported a "fear of the unknown" with regard to handling computers, an anxiety that telemedicine will lead to job loss, an apprehension that the initially high investment required is not viable, or a concern that the bedside presence of consulting physicians in local hospitals will decline (51, 57). Fear that the integration of new communication technologies into telemedicine systems may alter existing work practices, challenge physician referral methods, or interrupt workflow may also affect physician acceptance of telemedicine (17). Designing systems that enhance rather than dislodge current work practices and effectively communicating them to practitioners presents a challenge and an opportunity to ensure appropriate and meaningful uptake of telemedicine systems within low-income settings (65).

As with many other types of health care interventions, the lack of information available regarding legal policies, guidelines, or minimum standards concerning the use of telemedicine in the clinical context may also be preventing the adoption of such technologies.

### 2.2.3 Legal and ethical considerations for telemedicine in developing countries

Telemedicine progress can be better measured when legal frameworks are introduced, national eHealth policies are developed, more human resources are trained, regular funding is committed, and long-term plans are made (16). However, care must be taken to enact and enforce telemedicine in a way that does not hinder its progress or promise (67). Telemedicine, in general, must contend with many legal and ethical considerations, especially in the area of patient privacy and confidentiality. In the developing world, however, other issues have become more prominent.

Cross-border legalities are a concern for developing countries that use telemedicine services to connect with health professionals from more than one country. A crucial question that needs to be addressed in this scenario is: Which country's law applies or has jurisdiction over the service? (21). A host of problems can occur when the health laws of participating countries conflict. What happens if a mistake occurs? Who takes ultimate responsibility for the service and care provided? Unfortunately, these types of legal questions are insufficiently addressed by national health laws at present (69). Uncertainty may impact the use of such services in both industrialized and developing countries. Additionally, the lack of information about legal policies and guidelines concerning the use of telemedicine in the clinical context may be a deterrent to the adoption of such practices.

Ethically, the use of telemedicine services in developing countries has also been questioned. Clearly, using telemedicine in underserved countries to increase access to care brings great benefit; some question, however, whether this is the most effective use of scarce resources (34). In incidences where telemedicine services do improve overall health outcomes the value is high, but this can come at a great burden to a struggling health care system. Telemedicine may cost developing countries in other ways as well, such as placing high time demands on personnel and other resources like electricity.

## 2.2.4 Implications for telemedicine development, implementation, evaluation, and sustainability

An overall lack of evaluation data, trials, and published results concerning telemedicine initiatives in developing countries has limited the amount of evidence on the impact and effectiveness of telemedicine (41, 70). Regions may lack the expertise and funding to document experience with telemedicine and conduct research (16). Clinical outcomes are hard to document as sample sizes involved in telemedicine are often small and it is particularly difficult to obtain follow-up data from patients (23, 59).

While there is, overall, a paucity of rigorous research and evaluation that addresses all of the areas of population health outcomes, economic analyses, and patient/provider satisfaction, the variety of studies published in the peer reviewed literature shed light on opportunities, successes, challenges, and implications for telemedicine in developing countries. Evaluation is vital to systematically document best practices and lessons learnt from country-specific telemedicine networks. Such evaluations will show which networks demonstrably alter health outcomes, prove to be cost-effective and sustainable; these can then provide a model for other countries to adapt for their own contexts (14). Critical success factors identified in the literature include: setting clear programme goals; garnering government and institutional support; adapting existing user-friendly interfaces; determining accessibility and connectivity constraints; implementing standards and protocols; and disseminating evaluation findings (62, 71).

## 2.2.5 Key lessons from the literature

Health system transformation requires the involvement of all stakeholders. Partnerships usually facilitate change and the telemedicine sector is no different. Community leaders, health professionals, academic institutions and educators, health administrators, and policy-makers represent the best alliance to make changes necessary to reflect and react to societal needs. Figure 1 represents this principle.

Figure 1. Social accountability partnership pentagram

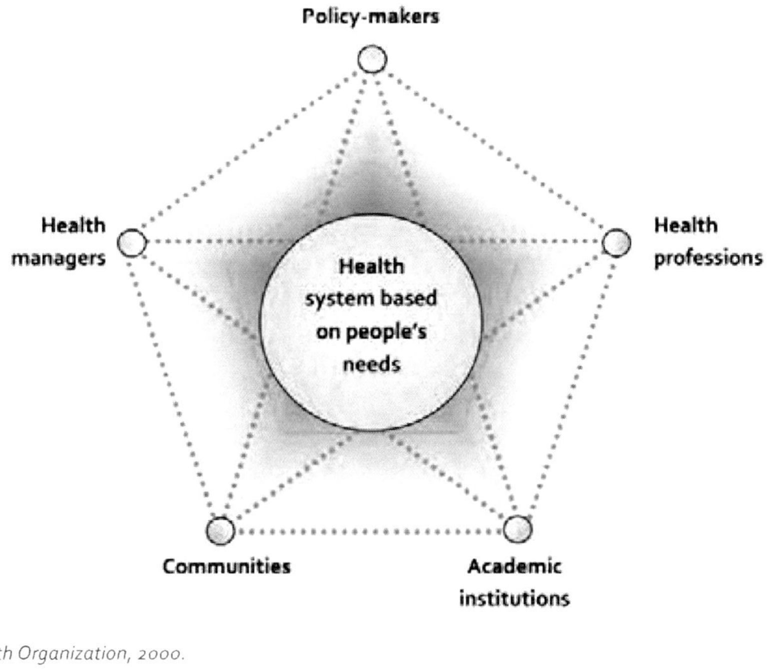

*Source: World Health Organization, 2000.*

Figure 1 shows five sectors, namely health policy, administration, academic institutions, health providers, and community. Vis-à-vis these sectors, telemedicine's development, implementation, evaluation, and sustainability in developing countries was reviewed during a thematic review of the literature. Five key lessons were drawn from this review, which inform social accountability in health practice across the sectors; they are described below.

**Lesson 1:** Collaboration, participation, and capacity building are fundamental to the success and sustainability of telemedicine initiatives.

Telemedicine is emerging as a cost-effective way for industrialized countries to aid in the capacity building of health care systems in the developing world. Modest investment in telemedicine can result in reductions in burden of disease, while increasing capacity of both referred specialists and referral sites (46). New channels for communication and collaboration have enabled the dematerialization of several processes usually hindered by deficient physical infrastructures (e.g. storage of patient data). To be most effective, however, strategies for integrating telemedicine initiatives into existing health systems require a collaborative approach, the identification of best practices, well-designed trials, and the incorporation of the many social factors that impact user adoption (32). Collaboration depends on local expertise and capacity, which in turn can increase the usage of telemedicine programmes; one drives the other through collaboration, improving reliability and sustainability of programmes.

While the institutional anchoring of telemedicine tools within national health care strategies has been deemed as key for success (55, 72), this must be done in conjunction with well-organized stakeholder collaboration. To be sustainable and to guarantee the reliability, security, safety, and timeliness for exchanging sensitive information, telemedicine services require the active participation of all users (38, 50). Education may be required to mitigate negative perceptions of telemedicine that hinder user acceptance and participation (73). The quality of telemedicine services may depend largely on the experts involved; experts should be therefore selected according to their expertise and commitment to delivering services via telemedicine (74). Finally, experts need to be committed to local capacity building, e.g. through train-the-trainer models and communities of practice linking champion-experts to mentor novices.

**Lesson 2:** Organizations and individuals engaging in telemedicine initiatives in developing countries need to be aware of the local context in which they work, i.e. available resources, needs, strengths, and weaknesses.

A major challenge facing international telemedicine initiatives designed to assist developing countries is the lack of a model appropriate to the realities of those settings. Differences in the needs and conditions between developing and industrialized countries make it imperative for telemedicine applications to be tailored to local contexts (39, 64). Variations in local resources, infrastructure, and personnel impose constraints on available medical services and influence the technical feasibility of certain telemedicine applications. To be technically feasible, telemedicine applications should be developed in parallel with that of ICTs and basic technological infrastructures and connectivity locally (34, 61, 66). Further, when collaborating internationally, it is essential that consulting health-care professionals are familiar with local protocols, facilities, resources, and expertise in order to suggest feasible and appropriate diagnostic and therapeutic plans (23, 34, 60). It is also imperative that such collaborations support and empower remote sites and foster sustainable ways to improve the capacity of consulting health care personnel, rather than replacing direct care by local health-care professionals (31).

ICT applications used in telemedicine have the potential to improve education, training, knowledge sharing, health research, and access to care throughout the world in culturally appropriate ways that address fundamental needs, as well as specific health needs in each country. The integration of sociotechnical issues and priorities into the design and implementation of telemedicine is a critical factor for success (2). While many telemedicine projects in developing countries represent international and national partnerships, it is vital for the priorities and processes of such collaborations to be informed locally. Support for mentoring relationships between new partnerships/initiatives and successful programmes, as modelled by the AMIA Global Partnership Program (71), not only builds capacity but also allows for reciprocal learning opportunities between partners in developing and industrialized regions.

**Lesson 3:** Use simple solutions that appropriately meet the needs of a clinical context or community to optimize cost-effectiveness and minimize complexity in change management.

Simple, user-friendly interfaces and systems that people with little to no technical expertise and limited English-language knowledge can operate are important means of overcoming barriers to implementation and enabling a swift diffusion of telemedicine applications in health care within developing countries (19, 48, 65). This principle is valid with technical solutions as well.

Simple, low-cost, low-bandwidth solutions have proven to be successful for delivering telemedicine in the developing world (19, 44). Store-and-forward e-mail, in particular, has shown to be a low-cost and useful application of telemedicine in a variety of specialties and international contexts not bound by bandwidth limitations (17, 45, 75, 76). Such success has challenged the notion that real time, high quality, videoconferencing is required for diagnostic assessment (77). Relatively low-cost Web-based conferencing, for example, can provide an engaging synchronous avenue to deliver education to health-care providers and facilitate dialogue between clinicians in industrialized and developing countries (53). Telemedicine applications by their very nature may be more cost-effective than other solutions to providing medical care (78). Evaluations of cost–benefit profiles have shown that networking resources using telemedicine programmes can be advantageous when compared to activities such as funded fellowship programmes or staff exchanges between institutions, or the building and maintenance of new hospitals and clinics (24, 78).

**Lesson 4:** Evaluation is vital for scalability, transferability, and continuing quality improvement of telemedicine; it should include documentation, analysis, and dissemination.

Considering the low-level of infrastructure and the limited financial resources in many developing countries, careful evaluation and planning of telemedicine is imperative; it should be conducted in order to optimize the use of available resources (41, 61). To make evaluation possible, participating sites need to ensure good medical record keeping that enables reporting on outcomes (23). Such evaluation can be used to inform the modification of pilot projects to achieve cost-effectiveness and scalability (23) as well as to assess the transferability of projects to other medical subspecialties and locations (79). Lessons learnt should be shared in order to improve future research and the development of telemedicine applications (80). Methodologically sound research studies are also required to generate reliable data for policy-makers (59).

There is a need for participatory models of research and evaluation that engage local stakeholders in the development, design, and implementation of contextually meaningful research questions, processes, and outcomes. This builds capacity at the local level for research and evidence that can support practice change at the individual level and inform policy and systems change at the macro level. Further, the principles of ownership, control, access, and possession (*81, 82*) of local processes and data contribute to adoption, and meaningful evaluation that responds to local constraints and strengths. An interdisciplinary approach is needed that attends to local needs, with all stakeholders contributing to the full picture. This includes clinical and public health outcomes (with health broadly defined), patient and provider satisfaction, and economic analyses that are able to monetize social benefit (*82*). Along with the implementation and dissemination of research and evaluation findings comes the ability for such findings to inform the development and adaptation of evidence-based policy and guidelines for telemedicine adoption across the various contexts found in developing countries (*63*).

Lessons can also be taken from the experiences of other countries. For example, experiences with telemedicine in India could have far-reaching benefits for poorer communities in developed countries as well as for developing countries (*62*). The reverse is also true: given that industrialized countries such as Australia, Canada, and the United Kingdom have begun to implement large health information systems that standardize and incorporate ICTs. They may be able to provide developing countries with valuable lessons to reduce the time and resources required to increase ICT utilization in health care (*68*). The question remaining is how best to ensure that knowledge is shared, and translated to practice in very different contexts. Partnerships between academics, health administrators, practitioners, policy-makers, and communities that entail reciprocal knowledge translation need to be supported through development and evaluation funding. Collaborative investments are essential to defining and meeting global eHealth challenges (*83*).

**Lesson 5:** The social benefits of telemedicine contribute to the health of communities and human development, and are important goals unto themselves.

Telemedicine has the potential to provide considerable humanitarian and development benefits by promoting access, collaboration, and resource sharing across jurisdictions (*66*). One of the documented examples of the realization of this potential, described by Wootton and colleagues (*84*), is the second-opinion consultation system operated by the Swinfen Charitable Trust. This global eHealth system has operated for altruistic, rather than commercial reasons, and also provides a context for global health professional education and evaluation. High standards of care can be maintained via telemedicine and quality of life can be improved, while sparing patients the need to travel long distances to reach hospitals or to consult physicians (*29*). Telemedicine may also provide additional levels of service to remote regions, such as elementary and secondary education and e-commerce, which can provide concomitant benefits and may have positive impacts on communities (*28*).

By facilitating collaboration, telemedicine endeavours can support the empowerment of remote sites, contribute to continuing health education, and extend communities of practice and support to health-care professionals in the developing world (*31, 85*). Telehealth and distance learning through the Internet may be one of the most effective pedagogical methods currently available. These methods allow the health workforce to consult specialists and to seek guidance through the use of e-mails while stationed at their posts (*37*). Continuous support of health-care professionals via training, discussion within communities of practice, and access to informational resources is an important step towards launching and sustaining telemedicine projects and programmes (*61, 86*).

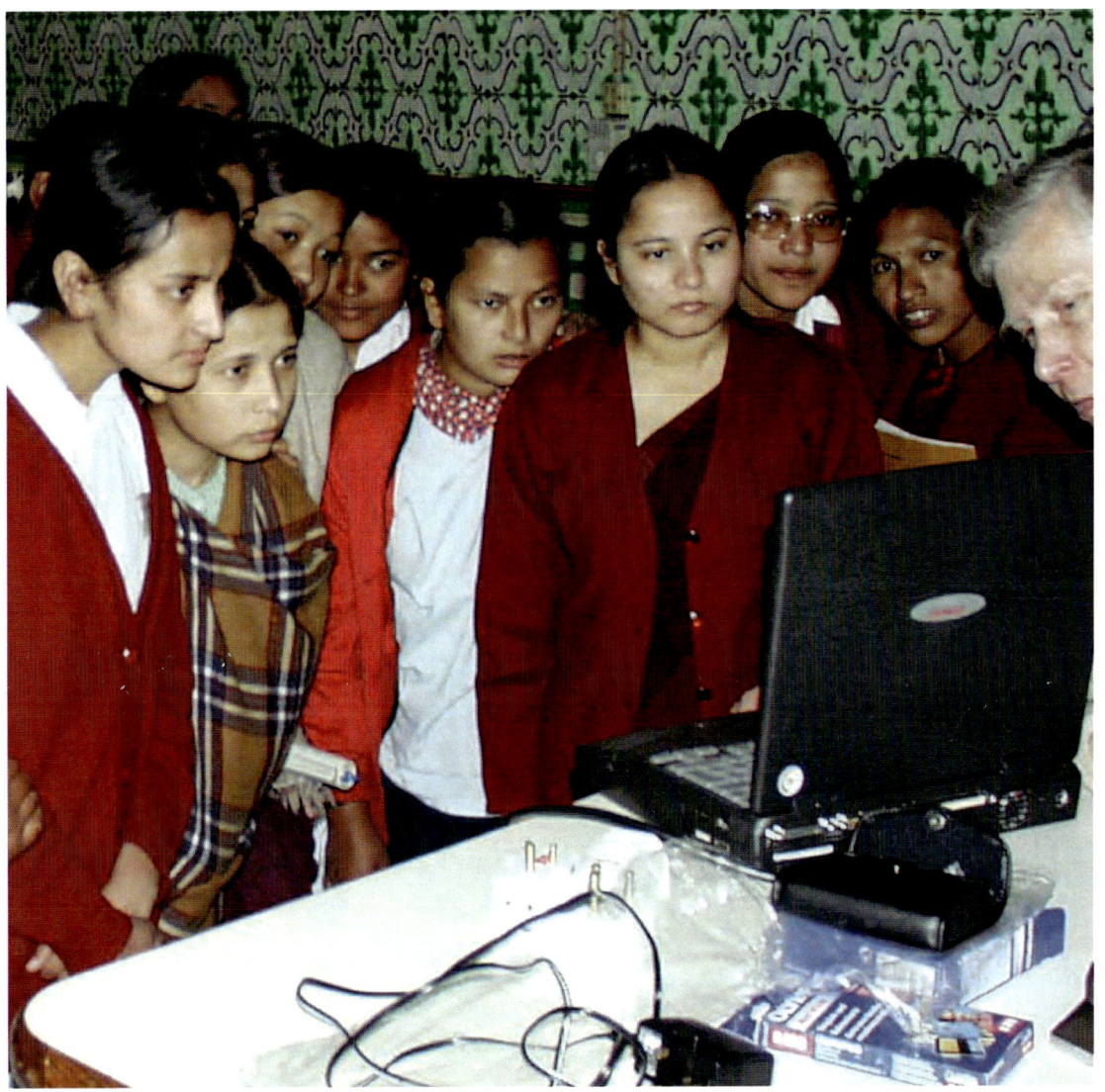

*Lord Swinfen providing an introduction to telemedicine at the Lalitpur Nursing Campus, Kathmandu (Photograph: Swinfen Charitable Trust)*

# 3 | GOe Second Global Survey on eHealth

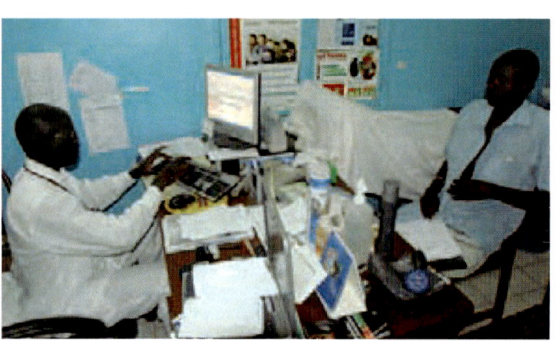
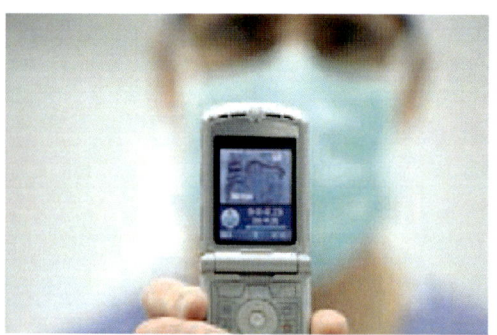
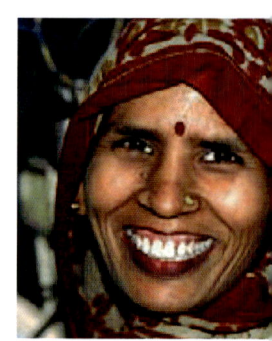

WHO's eHealth resolution adopted in 2005[1] focuses on strengthening health systems in countries through the use of eHealth; building public-private partnerships in ICT development and deployment for health; supporting capacity building for the application of eHealth in Member States; and the development and adoption of standards. Success in these areas is predicated on a fifth strategic direction: monitoring, documenting and analysing trends and developments in eHealth and publishing the results to promote eHealth uptake. In direct response to the eHealth resolution, the GOe was established to monitor and analyse the evolution of eHealth in countries and to support national planning through the provision of strategic information.

The first objective of the GOe was to undertake a global survey on eHealth to determine a series of benchmarks at national, regional, and global levels in the adoption of the necessary foundation actions to support the growth of eHealth. The aim was to provide governments with data that could be used as benchmarks for their own development as well as a way to compare their own progress with that of other Member States. In 2005 the GOe conducted a survey to compile those data.

The second global survey on eHealth was conducted in late 2009 and was designed to build on the knowledge base generated by the first survey. While the first survey was general and primarily asked questions about the national level, the 2009 survey was designed to be thematic with far more detailed questions used to explore areas particular to eHealth. The survey has provided the GOe with a rich source of data which is being used to create a series of eight publications – The Global Observatory for eHealth series – due for publication in 2010 and 2011.

1   WHA 58.28: http://apps.who.int/gb/ebwha/pdf_files/WHA58/WHA58_28-en.pdf.

Each publication in the series is primarily targeted at ministries of health, ministries of information technology, ministries of telecommunications, academics, researchers, eHealth professionals, nongovernmental organizations (NGOs) involved in eHealth, and donors.

## 3.1 Survey implementation

In creating the second survey, the GOe benefited from many of the lessons learnt from the first global survey: disseminating the instrument in digital format, working with WHO regional offices and Member States to encourage survey completion, as well as processing the data and analysing the results.

### 3.1.1 Survey instrument

The instrument focused on issues relating to processes and outcomes in key eHealth areas. Objectives for the survey were to identify and analyse trends in eight thematic areas (Table 1).

Table 1. Eight thematic areas addressed in the 2009 survey

| Theme | Action |
|---|---|
| mHealth | Identify the diverse ways mobile devices are being used for health around the world and their effectiveness. Highlight the most important obstacles to implementing mHealth solutions. Consider whether mHealth can overcome the 'digital divide'. |
| Telemedicine | Review the most frequently used telemedicine approaches worldwide as well as emerging and innovative solutions. Encourage the growth and acceptance of telemedicine globally, particularly in developing countries. |
| Management of patient information | Describe the issues relating to the management of patient information at three levels: local health care facility, regional/district, and national. Analyse the trends in transition from paper to digital records. Identify actions to be taken in countries to increase the uptake of digital patient records. |
| Legal and ethical frameworks for eHealth | Review the trends in the introduction of legislation to protect personally identifiable data and health-related data in digital format as well as the right to access and control one's own record. Identify and analyse the control of online pharmacies by Member States. Review actions of governments to protect children from harm on the Internet. |
| A systematic review of eHealth policies | Identify the uptake of eHealth policies worldwide and analyse them by WHO region as well as World Bank income group to establish possible trends. Systematically review the content and structure of existing strategies highlighting strengths and weaknesses. Propose model approaches for the development of eHealth policies including scope and content. |
| eHealth foundation actions | Review trends in the uptake of foundation actions to support eHealth at the national level including: eGovernment, eHealth, ICT procurement, funding approaches, capacity building for eHealth, and multilingual communications. |
| eLearning | Analyse the extent of use and effectiveness of eLearning among students and health professionals in the health sciences. |
| eHealth country profiles | Presentation of all participating Member States eHealth data aggregated by country to act as ready reference of the state of eHealth development according to selected indicators. |

### 3.1.2 Survey development

The survey instrument was developed by the GOe with broad consultation and input from eHealth experts. Planning for the 2009 global survey started in 2008 with the review of the 2005/2006 survey results and feedback from participating countries. One of the constraints identified in the first survey was the management of data and its availability for compilation and analysis. In order to facilitate data collection and management, Data Collector (DataCol)[2] was used to make the survey instrument available online, therefore streamlining the collection and processing of data.

A set of questions was developed and circulated in the first quarter of 2009 to selected partners in all regions through virtual teleconferences. Partners included those from government, WHO regional and country offices, collaborating centres, and professional associations. Over 50 experts worldwide were involved in the process. Collaborative efforts extended to other WHO programmes as well as international organizations such as the International Telecommunication Union (ITU) and the Organisation for Economic Co-operation and Development (OECD). An online forum to discuss the survey instrument and survey process was developed and hosted by the Institute for Triple Helix Innovation[3] based at the University of Hawaii at Manoa in the United States of America.

The GOe posted online a draft questionnaire for review by the partners, which was pilot tested in March 2009 in five countries: Canada, Lebanon, Norway, Philippines, and Thailand. The final version of the survey instrument was enhanced based on the comments and observations received following the pilot testing. To facilitate country response, the survey questions, instructions, and data entry procedures were translated into all WHO official languages and Portuguese.

### 3.1.3 Data collector

DataCol is a Web-based tool that simplifies online form creation for data collection and management and is designed, developed, and supported by WHO. The collected data are stored in an SQL database maintained by WHO database administrators, and can be exported as a Microsoft Excel file for further analysis using other statistical software.

This survey is the first time that DataCol has been used as the primary method of implementing an online survey of over forty pages of text and questions. Significant preparation and testing was required to ensure that the system was robust enough to accommodate the task.

The survey instrument and supporting documentation were categorized by language and entered into DataCol. Individual login names and passwords were assigned to each country to avoid multiple entries by the same country. Each participating country submitted a single national survey with input from a focus group of eHealth specialists. Country coordinators were responsible for completing the forms after obtaining agreement from the experts.

---

2  Web-based tool for online creation of forms in surveys developed by WHO.
3  http://www.triplehelixinstitute.org/.

## 3.1.4 Launching the 2009 survey

One of the most important tasks in executing an international survey is to build a network of partners at the regional level that can liaise directly with countries. To ensure the regional success of the 2009 eHealth Survey, all regional offices assigned staff to assist in coordinating the survey process and liaise with the Observatory in Geneva. Instructions for the survey procedures were circulated and then followed by a series of teleconferences. One significant outcome during the survey implementation was the development of strong working relationships with regional counterparts without whom it would not have been possible to successfully undertake such a task. Figure 2 shows the data collection process.

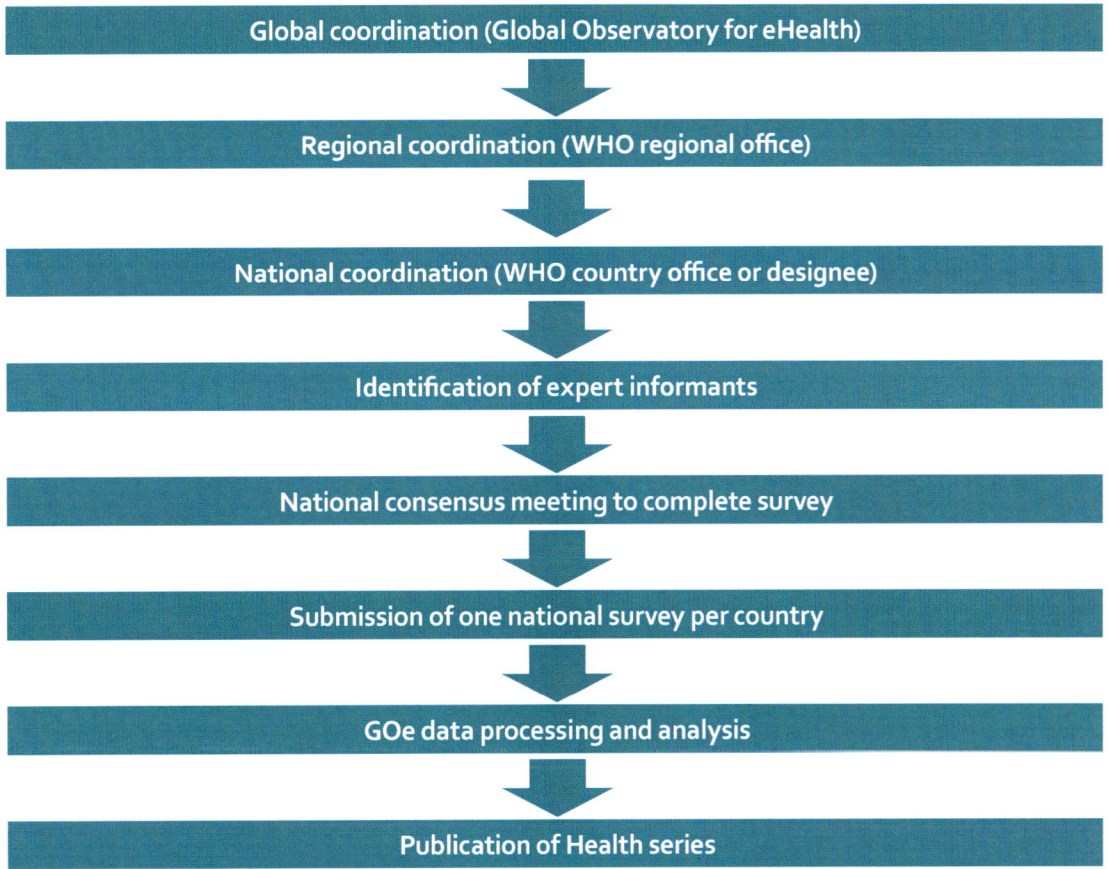

Figure 2. Data collection process for the 2009 eHealth Survey

The 2009 survey launched on 15 June 2009 and responses were accepted until 15 December. Regional focal points worked to encourage Member States to participate. In some cases this was easy; in others it required extensive discussions, not all of which were successful in achieving participation. Conducting a global survey is like conducting a campaign: the purpose and rewards of participation have to be conveyed to national coordinators and then to survey expert informants. It is important to build momentum and to maintain enthusiasm.

At the national level, coordinators were appointed to manage the task. Their responsibilities included finding experts in all the areas addressed by the survey, and organizing and hosting a full-day meeting where the survey would be completed collectively by the entire group. The number of expert informants ranged from 5 to 15 per country. While most countries entered their responses into DataCol, some countries preferred to send hard copies. GOe staff entered these responses into DataCol to ensure they were included in the data analysis.

### 3.1.5 Limitations

Member States were limited to one response per country; thus the expert informants were required to come up with a single response for each question that was most representative of the country as a whole. Coming to a consensus was difficult in cases where the situation varies widely within the country, or where there were significant differences in opinion. The survey does not attempt to measure localized eHealth activity at the subnational level.

The survey responses were based on self-reporting by the expert informant group for each participating Member State. Although survey administrators were given detailed instructions to maintain consistency, there was significant variation across Member States in the quality and level of detail in the responses, particularly to descriptive, open-ended questions. Also, while survey responses were checked for consistency and accuracy, it was not possible to verify all responses to every question.

The scope of the survey was broad, and survey questions covered diverse areas of eHealth, from policy issues and legal frameworks to specific types of eHealth initiatives being conducted in-country. Every effort was made to select the best national experts to complete the instrument; however, it is not possible to determine whether the focus groups had the collective eHealth knowledge to answer each question. Also, while the survey was circulated with a set of detailed instructions and terminological definitions, there is no guarantee that these were used when responding.

Finally, regional survey results should be interpreted with care. Results from the Region of the Americas and the Western Pacific Region, particularly, cannot necessarily be considered representative of the region as a whole; these regions had response rates and total number of responses below 50%. While the South-East Asian Region had the fewest number of responding countries, the region's response rate was the highest – the region consists of only 11 Member States. This should be considered when interpreting the results, as each responding country represents over 10% of the regional response.

For all regions, there was some degree of self-selection of the sample – Member States that have a high level of interest and/or activity in eHealth may have been more likely to respond to the survey than those with low levels of activity. This does not adversely impact the primary objectives of the survey, however, which were to document eHealth activity and trends around the world and to assess the level of eHealth development in participating Member States.

## 3.1.6 Data processing

On receipt of the completed questionnaires, all non-English responses were translated into English. Survey responses were checked for consistency and other errors, and countries were contacted for follow-up to ensure accurate reporting of results. Data were exported from DataCol in Microsoft Excel format and the data analysis was performed using R statistical programming language.[4] Data were analysed by thematic section: for closed-ended questions, percentages were computed for each possible response to obtain the global level results. In addition, the data were aggregated and analysed by WHO region and World Bank income group to see trends by these groupings (Table 2). Preliminary analysis based on aggregation by ICT Development Index[5] showed similar results as for those by World Bank income group; this is due to the high correlation between ICT Development Index and GDP per capita (Spearman $\rho=0.96$, $p<.001$). Therefore, these results were not included in this report. Cross-question analysis was performed where two or more questions were thought to be related, such as countries having introduced complementary policies, and the results were probed in greater depth as warranted. External health and technology indicators, such as mobile phone penetration, were introduced into the analysis for comparison purposes where relevant.

Results from the current survey were compared to those from the previous survey wherever possible; however, as the subject matter covered by the 2009 survey was considerably broader, and the survey questions were worded somewhat differently, there was little scope for this sort of analysis. In addition, the percentages in the 2009 survey were often not directly comparable, particularly at the regional level, as the sets of responding countries differed, as did the expert informants responding in each iteration of the survey.

Table 3. Response rate by WHO region

| Grouping | Advantage | Disadvantage |
|---|---|---|
| WHO region | WHO regional approach integrated into WHO strategic analysis, planning, and operational action. | Limited country commonality from an economic, health care, or ethnic perspective.<br>Less useful for other agencies or institutions wishing to interpret or act on GOe data. |
| World Bank income group | Clear economic definition based on GNI per capita.<br>Consistent application of criteria across all countries.<br>Simple four-level scale. | Does not account for income disparity, health of the population, or population age. |

*GNI, gross national income.*

---

4  http://www.r-project.org/.
5  http://www.itu.int/ITU-D/ict/publications/idi/2009/index.html.

## Response rate

Not all Member States completed all seven sections of the survey: 112 completed it entirely and 114 (59% of Member States; 81% of the world's population) completed at least one section (the Telemedicine Section). The response to the 2009 survey is roughly the same as for the previous global survey (58%), which is encouraging considering the 2009 survey instrument is significantly longer than that of 2005/2006. Figure 3 shows the countries that answered the Telemedicine Section of the survey. Tables 4 and 5 show the distribution of those countries by WHO region and World Bank income group, respectively.

Figure 3. Responding WHO Member States

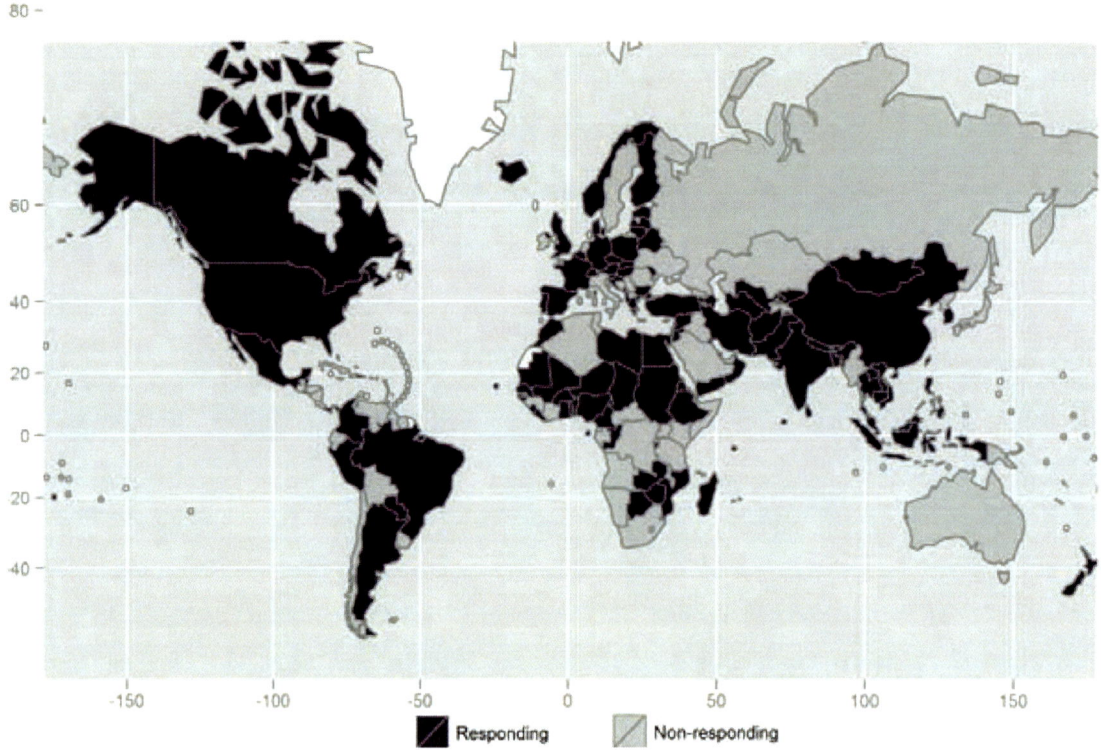

## Response rate by WHO region

Administratively, WHO is made up of six geographical regions. The regions are heterogeneous: Member States differ with respect to size, economy, and health care challenges. Nevertheless, it is still important to present high-level eHealth analyses at the regional level as this reflects the organizational structure and operational framework of WHO.

Table 3 shows considerable variation in country participation: for example responses ranged from 34% (in the Region of the Americas) to 73% (the South-East Asia Region). Numerous Member States indicated that they would not be able to participate in the 2009 survey due to resources being diverted to prepare and respond to the H1N1 pandemic, or due to other urgent public health issues arising from armed conflicts; this was the case with many countries from the region of the Americas. The Western Pacific Region has many small island Member States of which only a few responded to the survey, yielding a response rate of 48% for this region. The response rates for the Eastern Mediterranean, African and European Regions were over 60%. This was particularly encouraging for regions consisting of a large number of Member States such as the African and European Regions.

Table 3. Response rate by WHO region

|  | WHO region | | | | | |
|---|---|---|---|---|---|---|
|  | Africa | Americas | South-East Asia | Europe | Eastern Mediterranean | Western Pacific |
| Total number of countries | 46 | 35 | 11 | 53 | 21 | 27 |
| Number of responding countries | 31 | 12 | 8 | 36 | 14 | 13 |
| Response rate | 67% | 34% | 73% | 68% | 67% | 48% |

## Response rate by World Bank income group

The World Bank classifies all economies with a population greater than 30 000 into four income groups based on gross national income (GNI) per capita.[6] The classification is as follows: low income (US$ 975 or less); lower-middle income (US$ 976–3855); upper-middle income (US$ 3856–11 905); and high income (US$ 11 906 or more).[7] These income groups are a convenient and practical basis for analysis to look at trends in the survey results based on income level. Classification by income does not correspond exactly to level of development; however, low- and middle-income countries are sometimes referred to as 'developing' economies and high-income countries as 'developed' for convenience.

Table 4 shows the survey response rate by World Bank income group. Low-income countries had the highest response rate (70%), closely followed by high-income countries (63%). In terms of raw numbers, the distribution of responding countries was remarkably even, with 30 to 32 countries responding from the high-income, lower-middle income, and low-income groups; slightly fewer countries responded from the upper-middle income group.

Table 4. Response rate by World Bank income group

|  | World Bank income group | | | |
|---|---|---|---|---|
|  | High income | Upper-middle income | Lower-middle income | Low income |
| Total number of countries | 49 | 44 | 53 | 43 |
| Number of responding countries | 31 | 21 | 32 | 30 |
| Response rate | 63% | 48% | 60% | 70% |

---

6 http://data.worldbank.org/about/country-classifications.
7 based on country data from 2008.

# 4 Telemedicine results

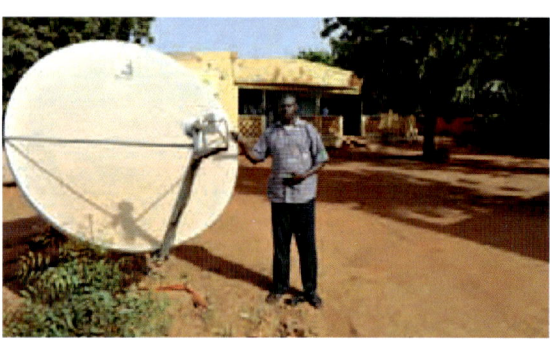 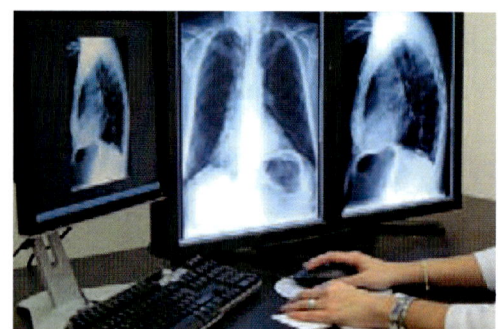 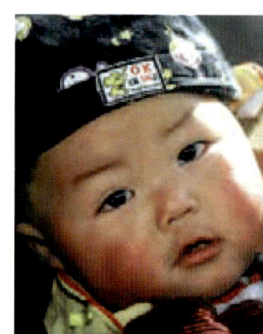

Analysis of the results of the Telemedicine Section of the second global survey on eHealth 2009 will follow in four areas:

1. Current state of telemedicine services;
2. Factors facilitating telemedicine development;
3. Barriers to telemedicine; and
4. Telemedicine information needs.

## 4.1 Current state of telemedicine services

To obtain an impression of the current state of telemedicine service provision, four of the most popular and established areas of telemedicine were surveyed specifically. Respondents were asked to indicate whether or not their country offered a service in each field, and if so, to give its level of development. Levels of development were classified as 'established' (continuous service supported through funds from government or other sources), 'pilot' (testing and evaluation of the service in a given situation), or 'informal' (services not part of an organized programme). The survey examined four fields of telemedicine:

- Teleradiology – use of ICT to transmit digital radiological images (e.g. X-ray images) from one location to another for the purpose of interpretation and/or consultation.
- Telepathology – use of ICT to transmit digitized pathological results (e.g. microscopic images of cells) for the purpose of interpretation and/or consultation.
- Teledermatology – use of ICT to transmit medical information concerning skin conditions (e.g. tumours of the skin) for the purpose of interpretation and/or consultation.
- Telepsychiatry – use of ICT for psychiatric evaluations and/or consultation via video and telephony.

> **KEY POINTS**
>
> - Teleradiology has the highest rate of established service provision across the four fields of telemedicine surveyed.
>
> - Provision of telemedicine is far less progressed in upper-middle, lower-middle and low-income countries than in high-income countries; this is the case for the proportion of countries with established services and the overall proportion of countries offering telemedicine services. Little difference was observed between upper-middle, lower-middle, and low-income groups with regard to the proportion of countries with established telemedicine services.
>
> - The African and Eastern Mediterranean Regions generally had the lowest proportion of countries with established telemedicine services, and a higher proportion of countries offering informal telemedicine services than other regions.

### 4.1.1 Telemedicine services globally

Teleradiology is currently the most developed telemedicine service area globally, with just over 60% of responding countries offering some form of service, and over 30% of countries having an established service (Table 5). While the proportion of countries with any form of service ranged from almost 40% for teledermatology and telepathology to approximately 25% for telepsychiatry, the proportion of countries with established services in those three areas was comparable at approximately 15%.

Table 5. Global implementation rates of telemedicine services

|  | Established | Pilot | Informal | No Stage Provided | Total |
|---|---|---|---|---|---|
| Teleradiology | 33% | 20% | 7% | 2% | 62% |
| Telepathology | 17% | 11% | 9% | 4% | 41% |
| Teledermatology | 16% | 12% | 7% | 3% | 38% |
| Telepsychiatry | 13% | 5% | 5% | 1% | 24% |

## 4.1.2 Telemedicine services by WHO region

Figures 4–7 provide an overview of teleradiology, telepathology, teledermatology and telepsychiatry services, respectively. They illustrate the proportion of countries with established, pilot, and informal services, grouped by WHO region. The global rates for each indicator are shown alongside the regional rates, for comparison.

While there was some variation across the four fields of telemedicine surveyed, the Regions of South-East Asia, Europe and the Americas generally had the highest proportion of responding countries with established services. The relatively high level of established teleradiology programmes appears to be driven by the South-East Asian and European Regions (75% and 50%, respectively); these two regions had a higher proportion of countries with established services than the global rate.

Conversely, the African and Eastern Mediterranean Regions consistently had the lowest proportion of countries with established telemedicine services. In the African Region, established services were reported in less than 10% of responding countries for all four of the telemedicine fields surveyed. In the Eastern Mediterranean Region, just over 25% of responding countries had established teleradiology services, while teledermatology and telepsychiatry programmes were established in less than 10% of countries; and not one country in the region reported an established telepathology service. In fact, services in these two regions were more likely to be informal in nature: in almost all cases the proportion of countries offering informal services was greater than the proportion with established services.

Figure 4. Teleradiology initiatives by WHO region

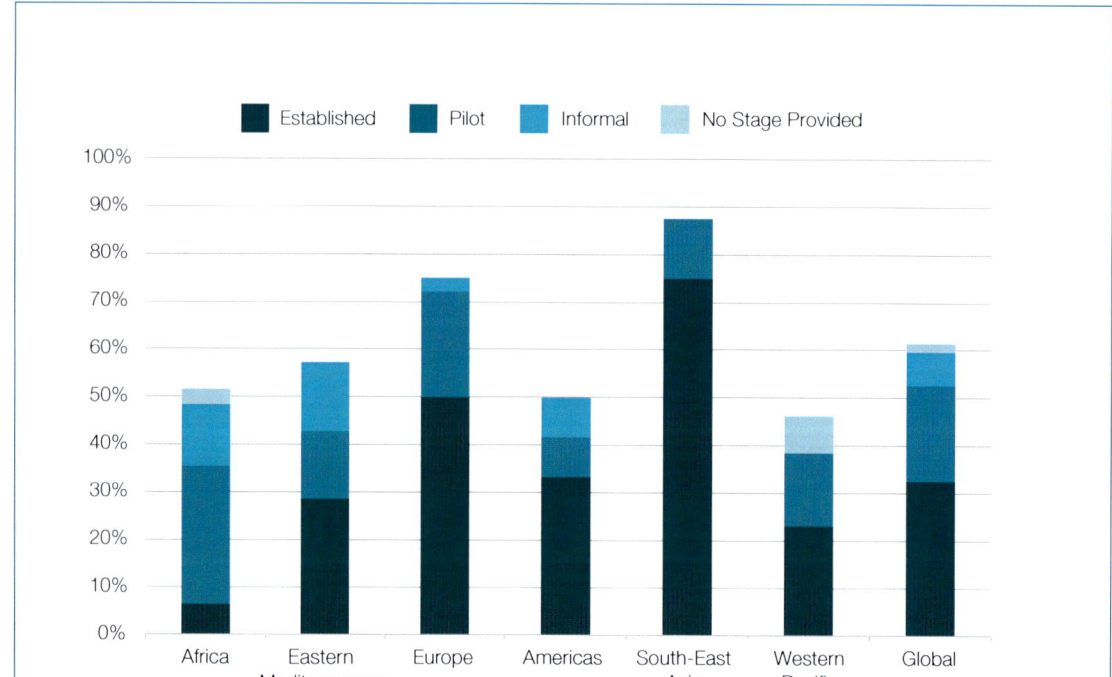

Figure 5. Teledermatology initiatives by WHO region

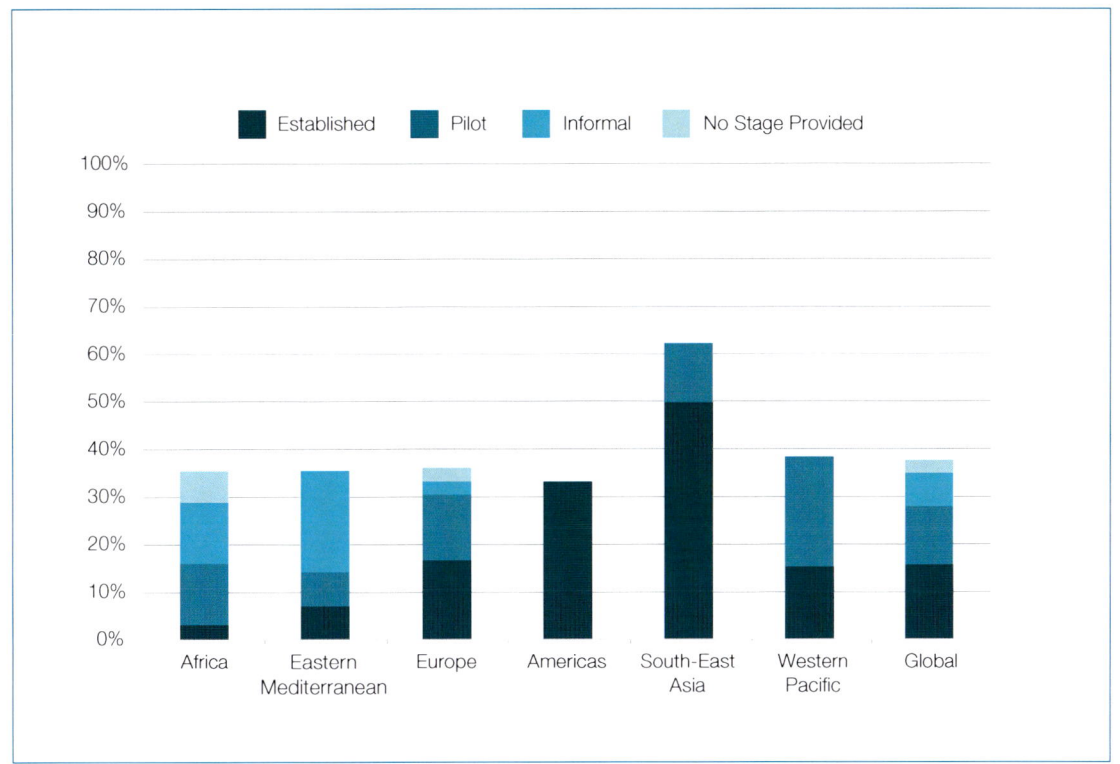

Figure 6. Telepathology initiatives by WHO region

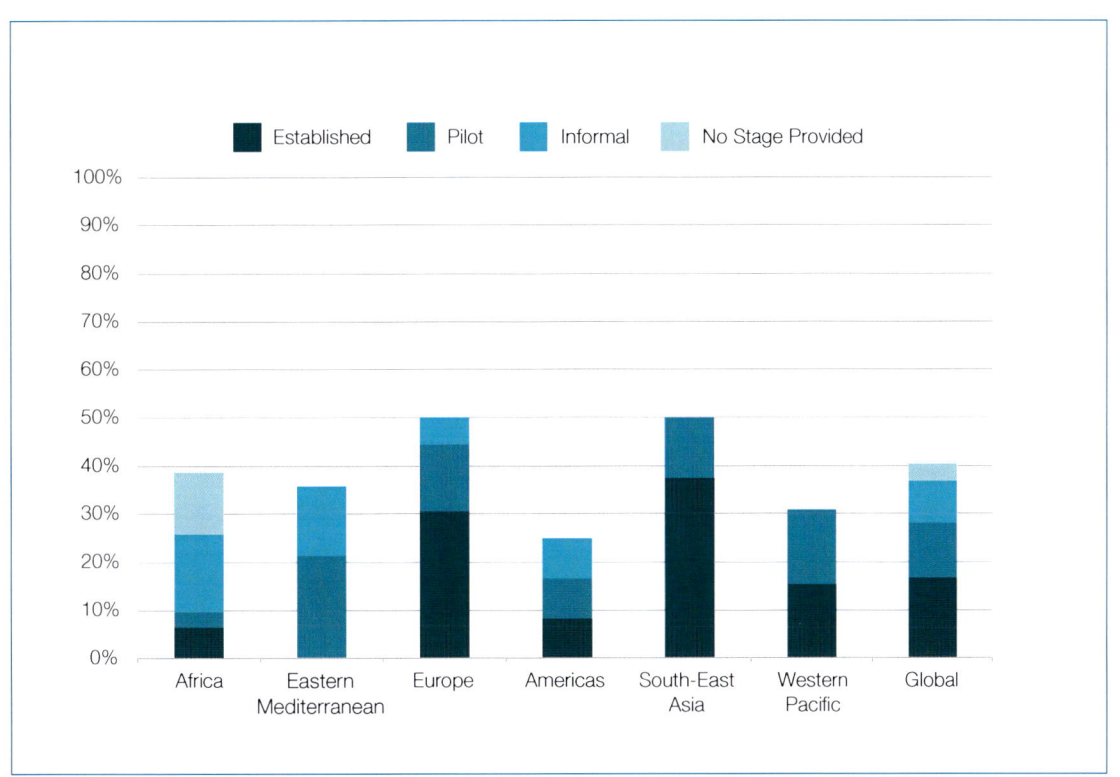

Figure 7. Telepsychiatry initiatives by WHO region

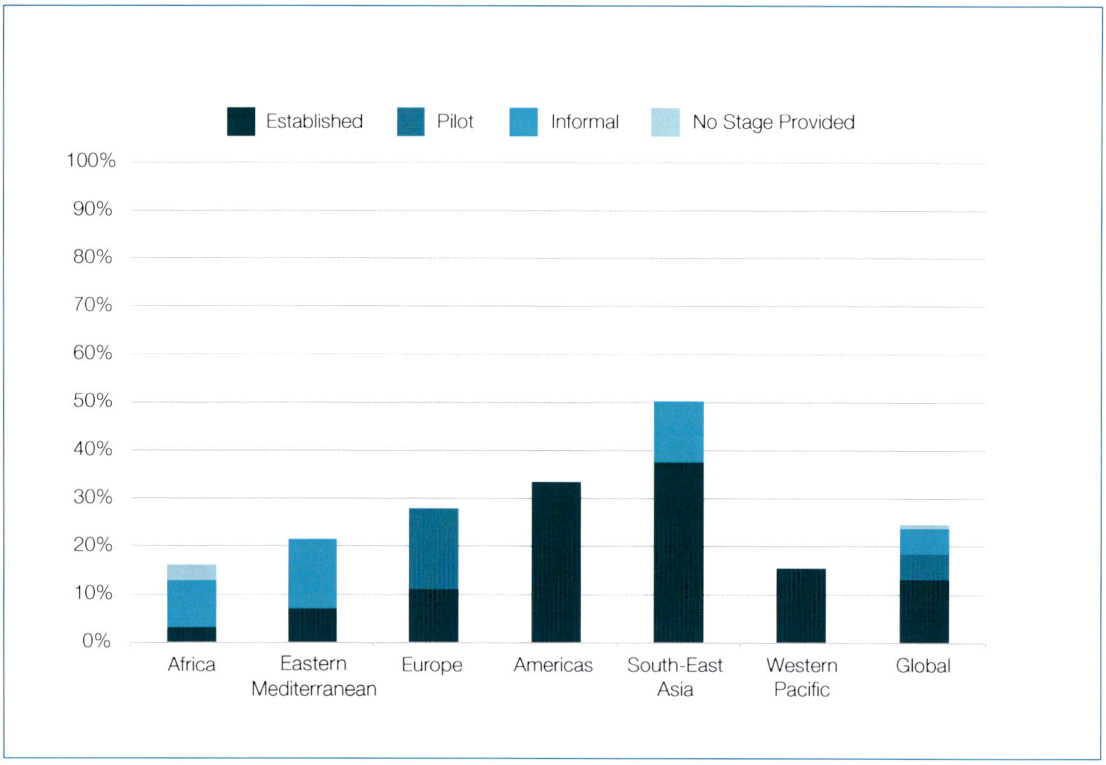

### 4.1.3 Telemedicine services by World Bank income group

Figures 8–11 illustrate the same results displayed by World Bank income group. These show that the percentage of countries with established services is considerably greater within the high-income group across all fields of telemedicine; the proportion of high-income countries with established services ranged from over 60% in teleradiology to 20% in telepsychiatry. High-income countries also reported the highest proportion of initiatives in the pilot stage, with the exception of teleradiology, which as shown is already quite well established in these countries. Among upper-middle, lower-middle, and low-income countries the proportion of countries with established, pilot, and informal initiatives is generally comparable within the four fields of telemedicine. While approximately 20% of countries in these three income groups reported established teleradiology services, the proportion of countries with established services was closer to 10% within the fields of telepathology, teledermatology, and telepsychiatry. Countries in the lower-middle and low-income groups were more likely to rely on informal telemedicine initiatives than were high and upper-middle income countries.

Figure 8. Teleradiology initiatives by World Bank income group

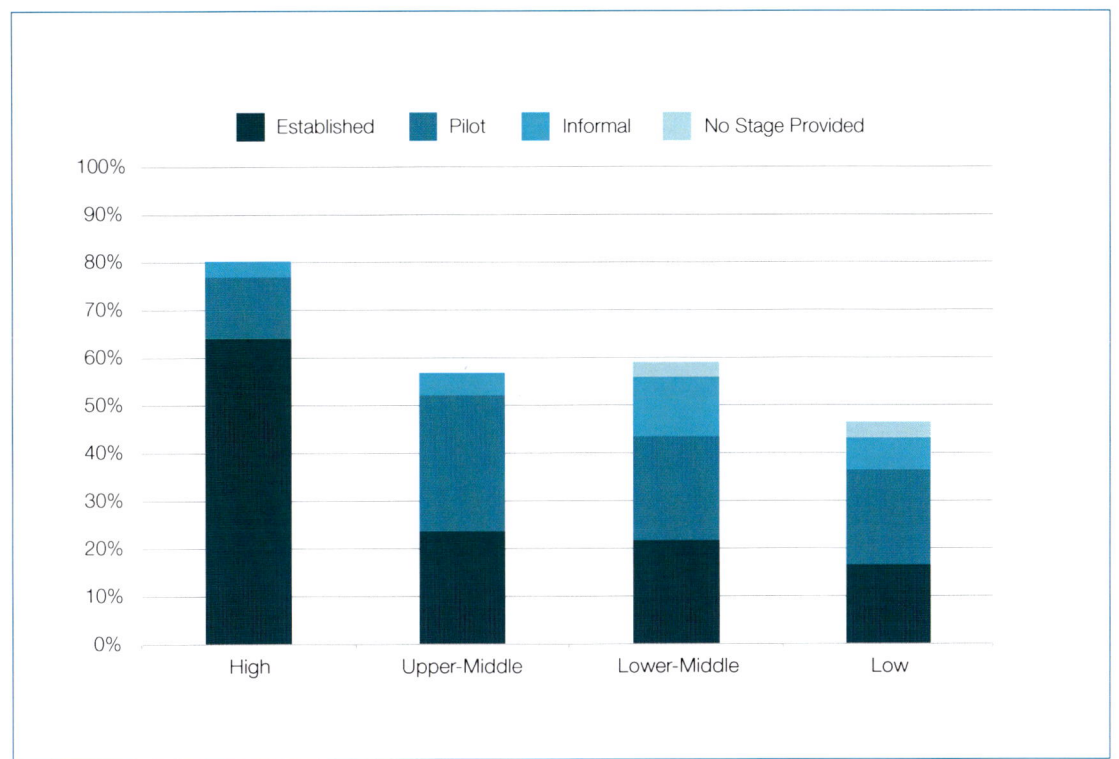

Figure 9. Teledermatology initiatives by World Bank income group

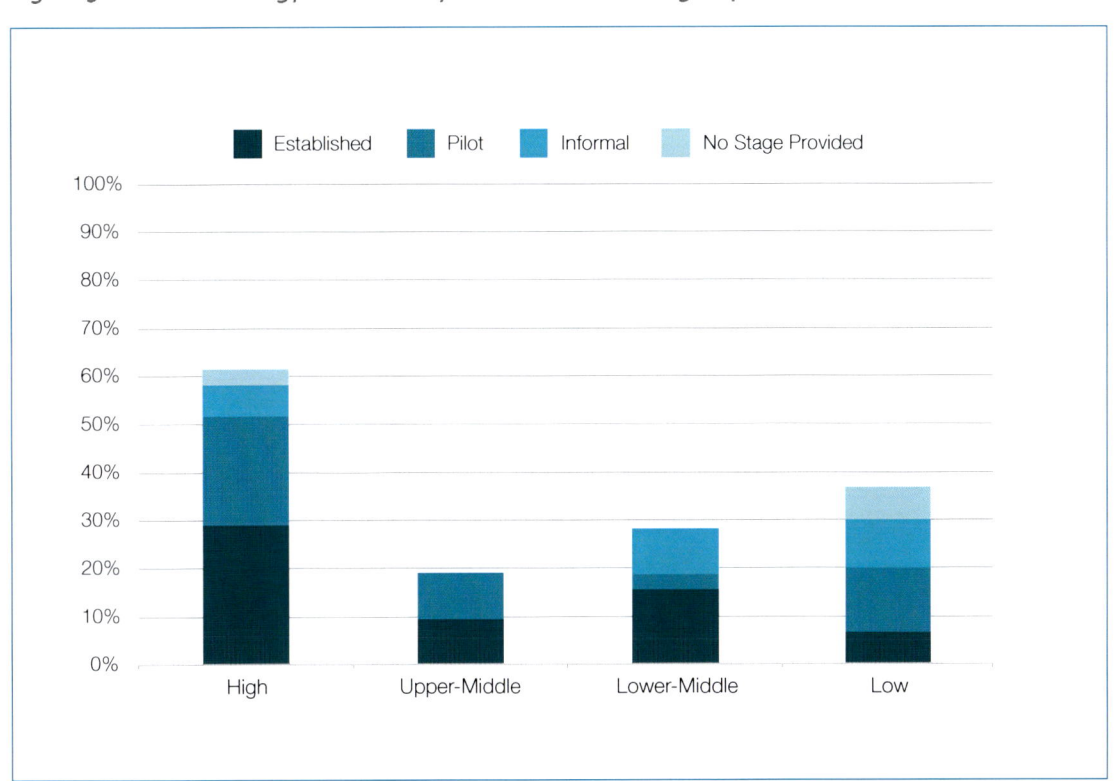

Figure 10. Telepathology initiatives by World Bank income group

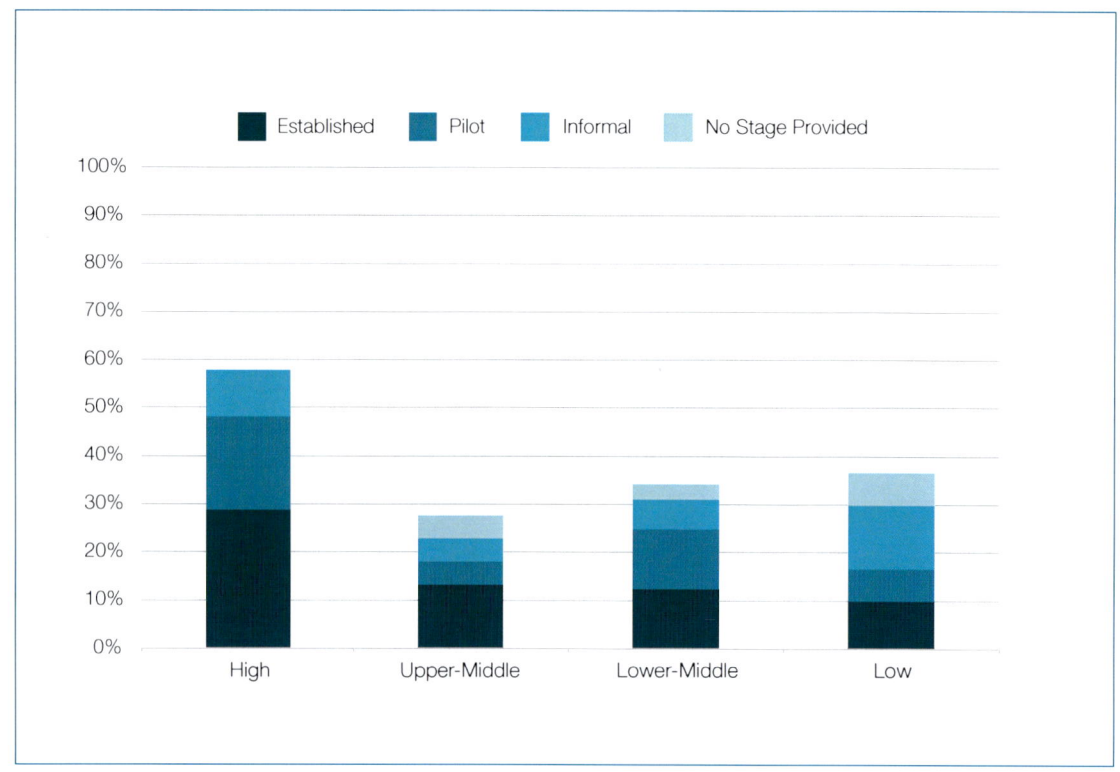

Figure 11. Telepsychiatry initiatives by World Bank income group

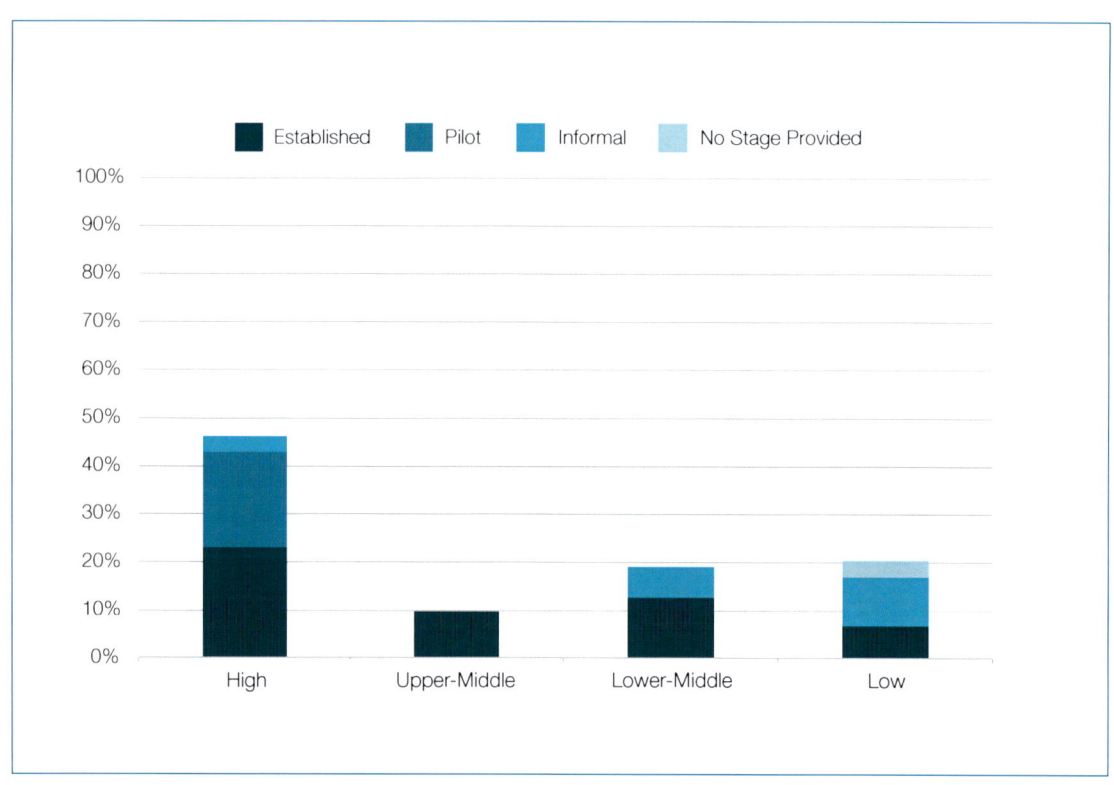

## 4.1.4 Other telemedicine initiatives occurring around the world

In an open-ended question, respondents were asked to list up to five additional telemedicine services currently offered within their country beyond the previous four fields surveyed above. Specifically, they were asked to describe the five most established or widespread services in their country. Responses to this, displayed in Table 6, illustrate the diversity of medical services currently being offered through telemedicine. Any service reported by two or more countries is represented; the full list of telemedicine services reported by responding countries, along with service providers, can be found in Appendix 1. The predominant service reported was cardiology and electrocardiography (ECG), with 28 individual countries providing these through telemedicine. Other relatively common services offered via telemedicine include ultrasonography, mammography, and surgery (as well as neurosurgery).

Note that countries were not asked to describe any one particular telemedicine service at this point. As such, these data are not directly comparable to the results presented above. Further, the services shown below may be underreported as respondents sought rather to highlight different and innovative examples of telemedicine being developed and used in their countries. Many diverse instances of telemedicine were reported as being in use by only a single country; some examples include emergency medicine, immunology, haematology, and speech therapy.

Table 6. Diverse telemedicine services offered by responding countries

| Telemedicine service | N°. of countries reporting service | Established | Pilot | Informal | No stage provided |
|---|---|---|---|---|---|
| Cardiology/Electrocardiography | 28 | 17 | 9 | 1 | 1 |
| Ultrasonography | 15 | 10 | 5 | 0 | 0 |
| Mammography | 12 | 8 | 4 | 0 | 0 |
| Surgery | 11 | 3 | 6 | 1 | 1 |
| Consultation | 7 | 5 | 1 | 0 | 1 |
| Ophthalmology | 6 | 2 | 2 | 2 | 0 |
| Nephrology | 5 | 4 | 1 | 0 | 0 |
| Obstetrics/Gynaecology | 5 | 3 | 2 | 0 | 0 |
| Diabetes | 4 | 2 | 1 | 1 | 0 |
| Patient monitoring | 4 | 0 | 3 | 0 | 1 |
| Paediatrics | 3 | 3 | 0 | 0 | 0 |
| Home care | 3 | 1 | 2 | 0 | 0 |
| Neurology | 3 | 1 | 2 | 0 | 0 |
| Neurosurgery | 3 | 1 | 1 | 0 | 1 |
| Stroke treatment | 2 | 2 | 0 | 0 | 0 |
| Urology | 2 | 2 | 0 | 0 | 0 |
| Oncology | 2 | 1 | 0 | 0 | 1 |
| Otolaryngology | 2 | 1 | 0 | 0 | 1 |

The examples in Table 6 highlight the range of data and information transmitted through ICTs for medical treatment and education. Services may be as minimal as the 'store-and-forward' transmission of relatively simple information such as ECG data or the e-mailing of digital mammography imagery or patient medical information for consultation purposes. But where infrastructure and bandwidth permits, the real-time transmission of detailed patient information and imagery, such as for ultrasonography and remote surgery, is also being utilized.

One result of particular interest was the significant number of countries that reported using telemedicine to provide cardiology and ECG services. Case study 3 provides an example from Norway. Figures 12 and 13 display the proportion of these countries by WHO region and World Bank income group, respectively. The African and Eastern Mediterranean Regions again had the lowest proportion of countries reporting telecardiology services, while services were generally more prevalent among high- and upper-middle income countries.

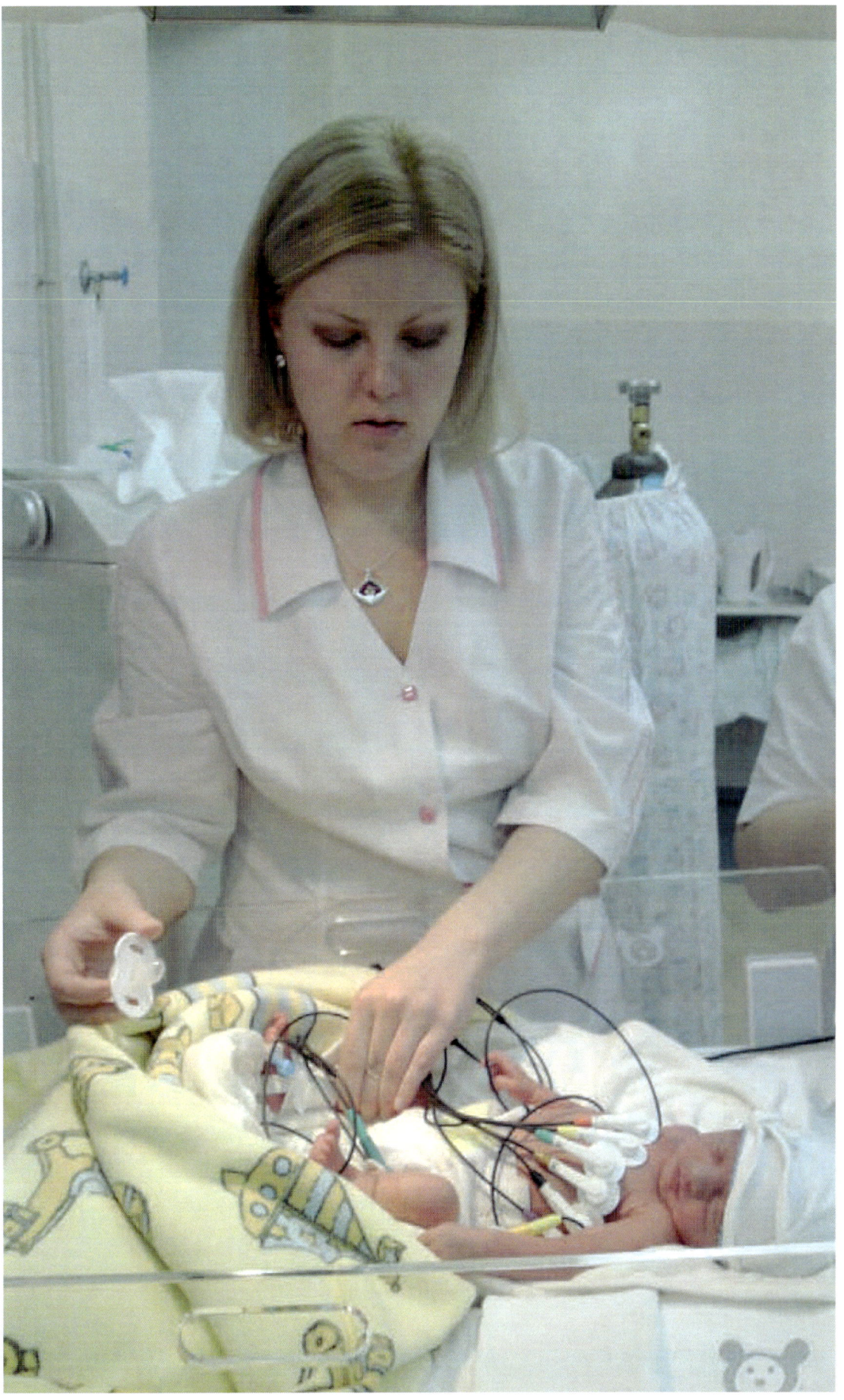

*Tele-ECG for neonatal intensive care units (emergency teleconsultations with cardiologists and cardiosurgeons in case of premature congenital heart abnormalities).*

*Photograph courtesy of Professor A. Vladzymyrskyy, Association for Ukrainian Telemedicine and eHealth Development, www.telemed.org.ua.*

# Norway's teleECG initiative

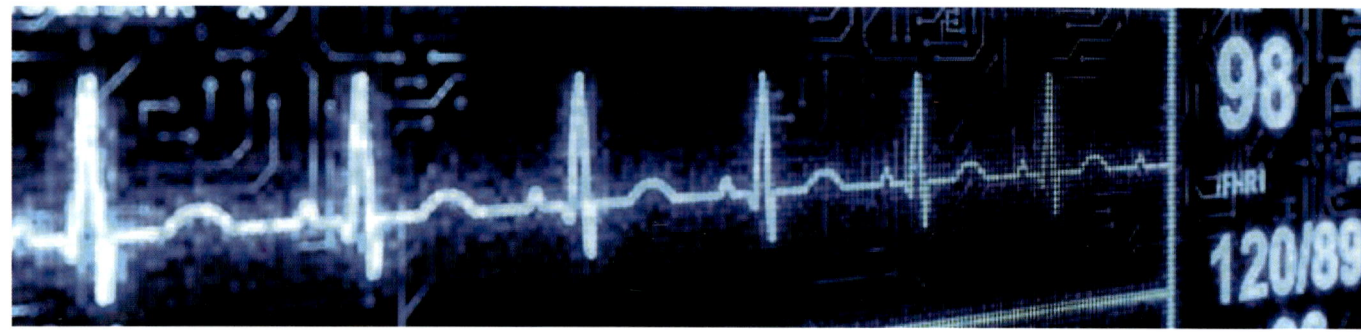

The teleECG initiative in Norway is a telemedicine service used to facilitate early diagnosis and treatment of suspected myocardial infarction in patients not in hospital. One of the first major telemedicine programmes in Norway, the teleECG initiative started in 1995 after initial pilot projects. Beginning in northern Norway as a way to reduce time from acute cardiac illness to treatment, teleECG is now available in over 100 ambulances and offered throughout the country with plans for all districts to offer it within the next 5–10 years.

This TeleECG system can either be used inside of the patient's home or in the ambulance en route to the hospital. Ambulances are fitted with equipment to capture and transmit ECG images to hospitals that have an image receiver and storage system for the images sent. Once received, the images are analysed by a cardiologist at hospital who is able to make a diagnosis and recommend an immediate course of action. While the equipment is mostly used for spot electrocardiograms, paramedics occasionally use it as a 12-point EKG.

This initiative has spurred radical changes. The teleECG system has helped decrease call time to treatment time, resulting in faster treatment and better patient outcomes. Cardio patients' outcomes have improved 15–20%. Having the ability to connect and consult with a cardiologist remotely has improved the quality of service and care from ambulances and paramedics. (It is estimated that approximately 50% of anti-thrombolytic treatment is now administered by paramedics.). The mobility of this service brings care to the patient.

The teleECG initiative has also improved cooperation between health professionals on an inter-professional team. Through experiences and challenges while participating in the teleECG system, paramedics, general practice physicians and cardiologists have learnt to work together more efficiently, which was a challenge at the initiative's outset.

Part of that challenge also involved legal discussions about the role and responsibility each health professional (the paramedic, general practice physician, and cardiologist) assumes during each event. While the training for this initiative has given paramedics more responsibility, it is ultimately the general practice physician (if on scene) who take full responsibility for the care of the patient. The consulting cardiologist at the hospital is responsible for the advice given. All three professionals are required to document the proceedings of the entire event (from diagnosis to treatment) for legal and security reasons.

A further challenge was training paramedics in the use of the equipment. What started as local courses and a supplementary CD to help familiarize and train the paramedics to use the teleECGs has now become a course fully integrated into their training, considerably expanding their skill set.

To fund the initiative, participating hospitals made the initial long-term investment in the equipment needed for the service. Since then, it has received basic hospital funding for maintenance. Remuneration for the health professionals involved differs. Because general practice physicians work privately, they are paid a fee per patient according to the intervention. However, both the paramedics and cardiologists are government funded. During an event, it has been agreed that whoever (the paramedic or general practice physician) initiates the treatment gets paid. The Danish Government provides ongoing funding support of the teleECG initiative.

This initiative is a cooperative effort involving ambulance services (government), general practice physicians (private), and the emergency department and cardiologists at hospitals (government); it is being expanded countrywide.

Acknowledgements
Mr Oddvar Hagen, Telemedicine Consultant
Norwegian Centre for Integrated Care and Telemedicine (NST)

Figure 12. Telecardiology initiatives by WHO region

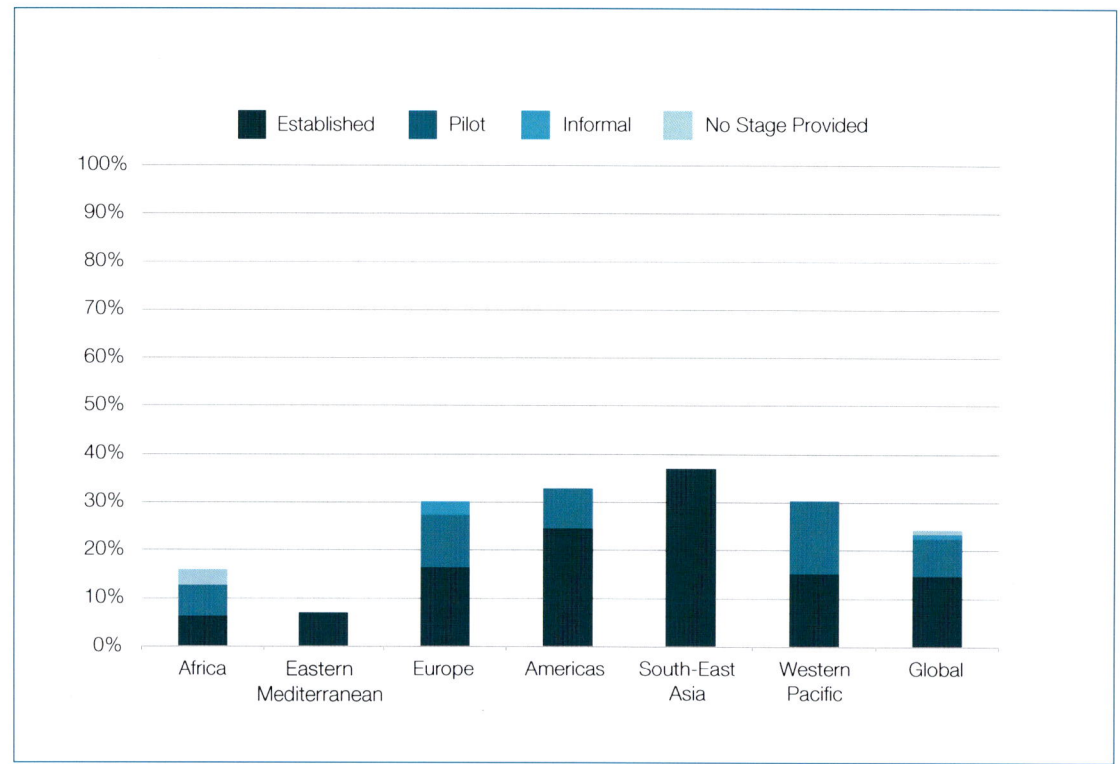

Figure 13. Telecardiology initiatives by World Bank income group

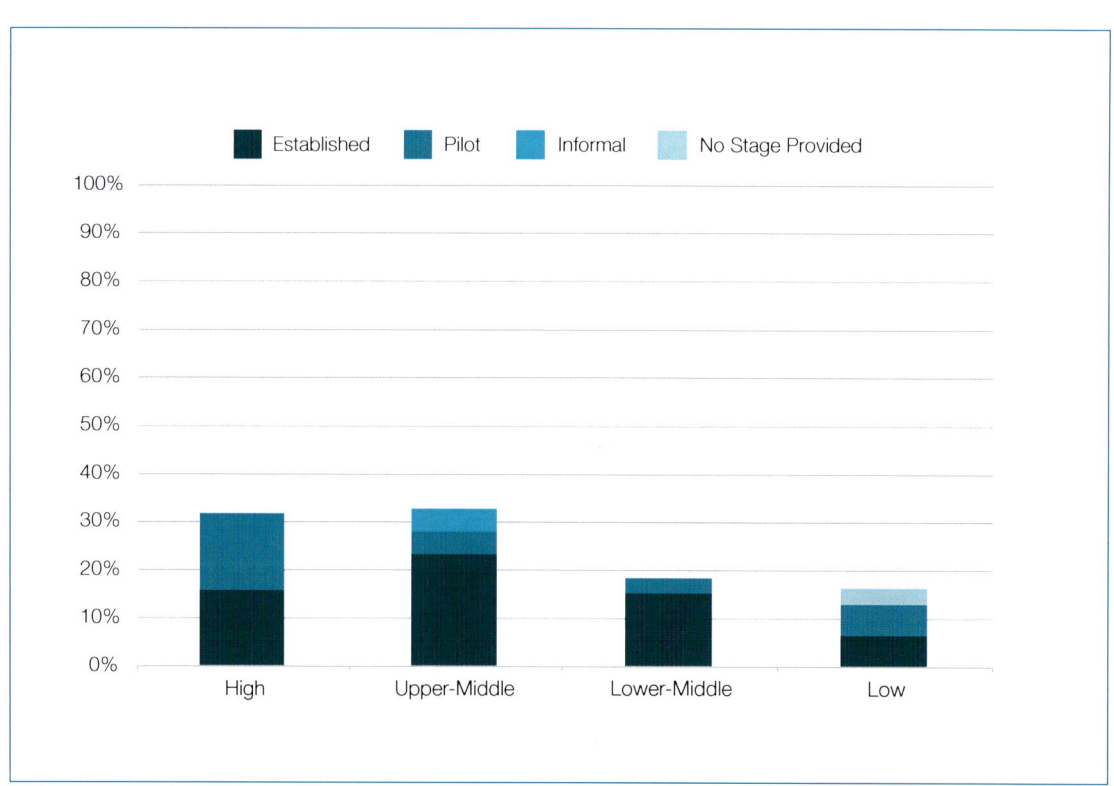

## 4.1.5 Implications for telemedicine services

The results of the survey show a consistent pattern between income group and the establishment of telemedicine services. At present, the vast majority of established services are found within the highest income countries. This is particularly evident in the field of teleradiology – generally considered to be the branch of telemedicine that has been best integrated into regular clinical practice. Furthermore, the majority of telemedicine development in the near future will likely occur in high-income countries, as suggested by the high proportion of countries with services in pilot stages of development.

The disparity between high-income countries and the rest of the world in telemedicine establishment may reflect the extent to which the implementation of, and capacity for telemedicine solutions are constrained by local resources and infrastructure. The most economically-developed countries generally have a sufficiently advanced information technology and communication infrastructure, greater freedom in their allocation of resources within the health care system, and more support for experimentation and research into new approaches to health care. This creates the capacity to develop and implement telemedicine solutions in a more formalized and systematic manner. In contrast, where countries outside of the high-income group do have telemedicine initiatives in place they are more likely to be informal in nature (i.e. not part of a structured telemedicine programme), such as connecting local health-care providers to specialists and consultative health care institutions.

The degree to which a telemedicine service has been established is often highly dependent on the complexity of the information being transmitted. Store-and-forward approaches are the most formalized initiatives; they are relatively simple to implement, require basic infrastructure and are generally not disruptive to traditional workflows of health professionals and patients. The store-and-forward approach is used predominantly in three of the four telemedicine services examined: teleradiology, telepathology, and teledermatology. The final service surveyed, telepsychiatry, was the least commonly reported; perhaps because it requires more real-time, bandwidth-intensive data transfer such as videoconferencing for consultations.

The broad range of telemedicine services employed outside of those four areas (Table 6) highlights not only the diverse and versatile nature of telemedicine, but the range and scalability of data and information that can be transmitted for the purposes of medical treatment, education, and consultation. There would be value in studying whether telemedicine services that cause less disruption to established health professional workflows (e.g. store-and-forward e-mails) are systematically more likely to be adopted than those that do (e.g. remote surgery), and whether this is due to disruption of workflow or to high ICT costs.. It would furthermore be instructive to monitor the adoption of simpler telemedicine applications to determine if that could lead to downstream adoption of more complicated telemedicine services. If so, it would suggest a progressively rising comfort level of technology adoption and acceptance.

Genuine questions remain as to whether telemedicine provides the most cost-effective solution in areas where resources are scarce and simply meeting the basic health needs of the population is of utmost priority, as is the case in the majority of developing countries. Although there is currently a conspicuous difference in the level of telemedicine implementation between high-income and low-income countries, it is encouraging to note the desire in some developing countries to implement telemedicine solutions at an informal level (i.e. using telemedicine services in an ad hoc fashion), particularly within the African and Eastern Mediterranean Regions. Such a desire illustrates recognition of the potential for telemedicine to make a positive impact on health care in the developing world, provided the right conditions are present. That these initiatives are still at an informal level could reflect the fact that to be technically feasible they must be scaled to parallel the available infrastructure and ICT capacity. When resources such as electricity, access to communication systems, or personnel are scarce, telemedicine initiatives should use these resources as efficiently as possible.

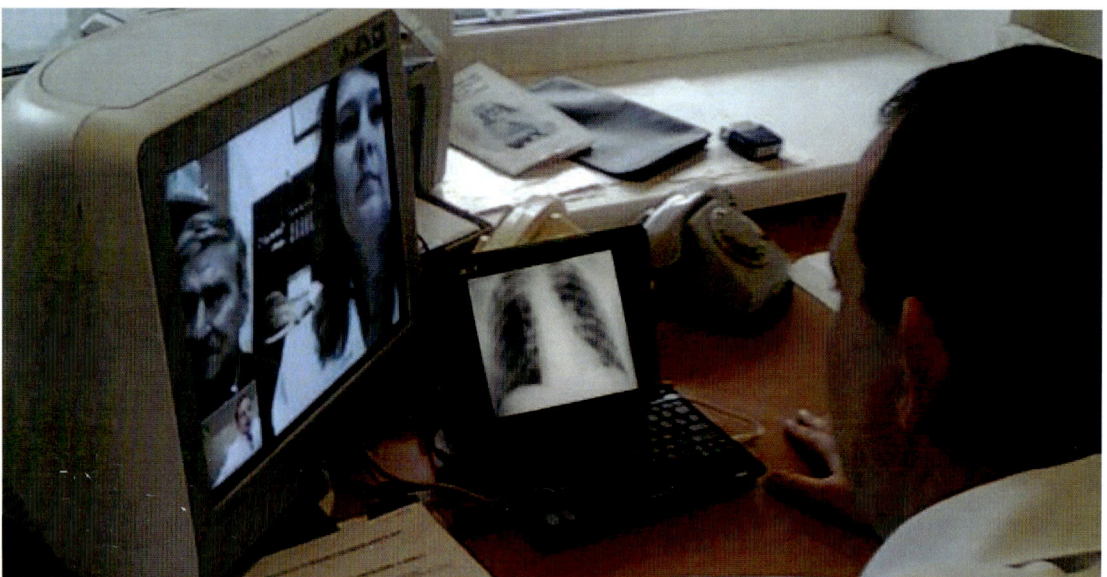

*Videoconference to provide expert second opinion.*

Photograph courtesy of Professor A. Vladzymyrskyy, Association for Ukrainian Telemedicine and eHealth Development, www.telemed.org.ua.

## 4.2 Factors facilitating telemedicine development

The survey examined progress made by countries with regards to some of the mechanisms that enable and facilitate the implementation of telemedicine technologies and solutions. The particular mechanisms included in the survey were:

- governance
- policy or strategy
- scientific development
- evaluation.

### KEY POINTS

- Approximately 30% of responding countries have a national agency for the development and promotion of telemedicine and its applications.

- Low- and middle-income countries appear as likely to have a national agency for telemedicine as high-income countries.

### 4.2.1 Governance

The planning and implementation of eHealth services requires complex and extended intersectoral collaboration, with stakeholders often coming from diverse backgrounds and with a range of priorities and agendas. Establishing sound governance mechanisms is advisable to help facilitate effective and transparent collaboration, necessary to successfully implement telemedicine services. Governing bodies have significant input into establishing telemedicine policy, and developing the required legal frameworks to deal with issues such as confidentiality, liability, and cross-border jurisdiction. Once telemedicine services are implemented, regulatory bodies are required to monitor and accredit practitioners. In many instances, however, need dictates that eHealth and telemedicine initiatives are initiated prior to governance mechanisms.

A good example of such a governing or regulatory body is a national agency focused on the development and promotion of telemedicine and its applications. When asked if their country had such an agency, approximately 30% of all responding countries reported that they did. These agencies varied considerably in scope, ranging from those with a very broad perspective, such as national ministries of health and university medical centres, to institutions focused on the development of ICTs, eHealth solutions, or specifically telemedicine applications.

Figure 14 gives an overview of the incidence of national telemedicine agencies of responding countries by WHO region. While the results showed some familiar trends – the South-East Asian and European Regions had the highest proportion of countries with a national telemedicine agency (approximately 50% and 40%, respectively) – the differences between regions were not pronounced, with the proportion of countries with telemedicine agencies ranging from 20% to 35% across the other regions.

Figure 15 provides an additional perspective, displaying the same countries by World Bank income group. Although it may have been expected that higher-income countries would be more likely to have a national telemedicine agency than lower-income countries, the results suggest there is no clear relationship between a country's income level and the establishment of a national agency for telemedicine.

Figure 14. National telemedicine agencies by WHO region

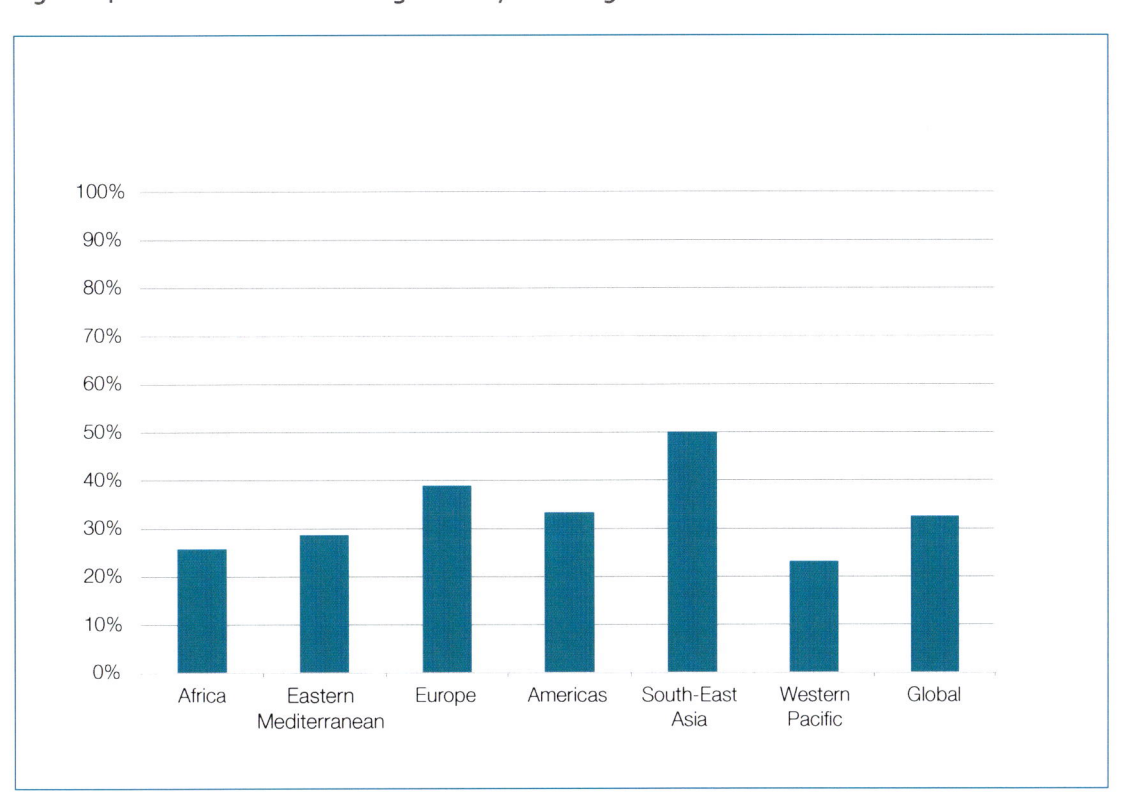

Figure 15. National telemedicine agencies by World Bank income group

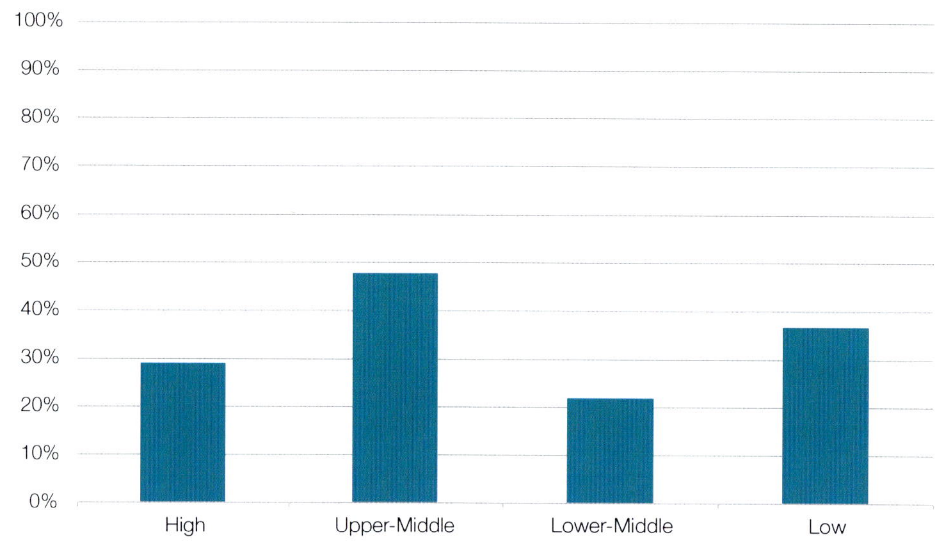

## Implications for governance

Obtaining governmental and institutional support can be a critical factor in the success of telemedicine, but as noted in the literature review in Section 2, even within developed countries little has been done to institutionalize telemedicine at a national level. The survey results support this, with two out of every three responding countries lacking a national telemedicine agency for the development and promotion of telemedicine and its applications. This may reflect a need for knowledge or evidence on the benefits of telemedicine, a perception that the benefits of telemedicine are insufficient, or a lack of demand from citizens or health-care professionals in these countries. A significant amount of work would be required to establish governance mechanisms to facilitate development of policy and national legal frameworks, but as noted previously, this could assist with the adoption and integration of telemedicine into health care systems and services.

### 4.2.2 Policy and strategy

Telemedicine policies and strategies can be used to outline the visions and objectives regarding the application, provision, control, standards, and ethics related to the national and international use of telemedicine solutions. Such policies may help facilitate and enable telemedicine adoption, potentially increasing the chance of successful implementation by providing a framework and protocol for the planning and development of services, as well as a standard by which the progress and results of telemedicine services can be better assessed.

## KEY POINTS

- Globally, 25% of responding countries reported that their country had a national telemedicine policy or strategy.

- Only 20% of responding countries reported having fully implemented or begun implementation of a national telemedicine policy or strategy.

- Developed countries are more likely than developing countries to have, or to have begun implementing a national telemedicine policy or strategy; however, significant growth in this area is forecast for developing countries.

- The African, Eastern Mediterranean, and South-East Asian Regions currently show the lowest rates of national telemedicine policy implementation, but the highest projected growth. These regions may require extra support in the development of telemedicine policies and strategies in the near future.

Respondents were asked whether their country had a national telemedicine policy or strategy. For the purpose of this report, the terms 'policy' and 'strategy' are used interchangeably. Figure 16 illustrates the results. A quarter of responding countries reported that they did have such a policy, although the examples provided by countries varied greatly in their depth and scope. The majority provided policy documents outlining general eHealth policies, and some documents outlining ICT use without providing information on specific applications. Few countries provided a document that specifically addressed policies or strategies for telemedicine implementation and use.

Figure 16. Countries reporting national telehealth policies

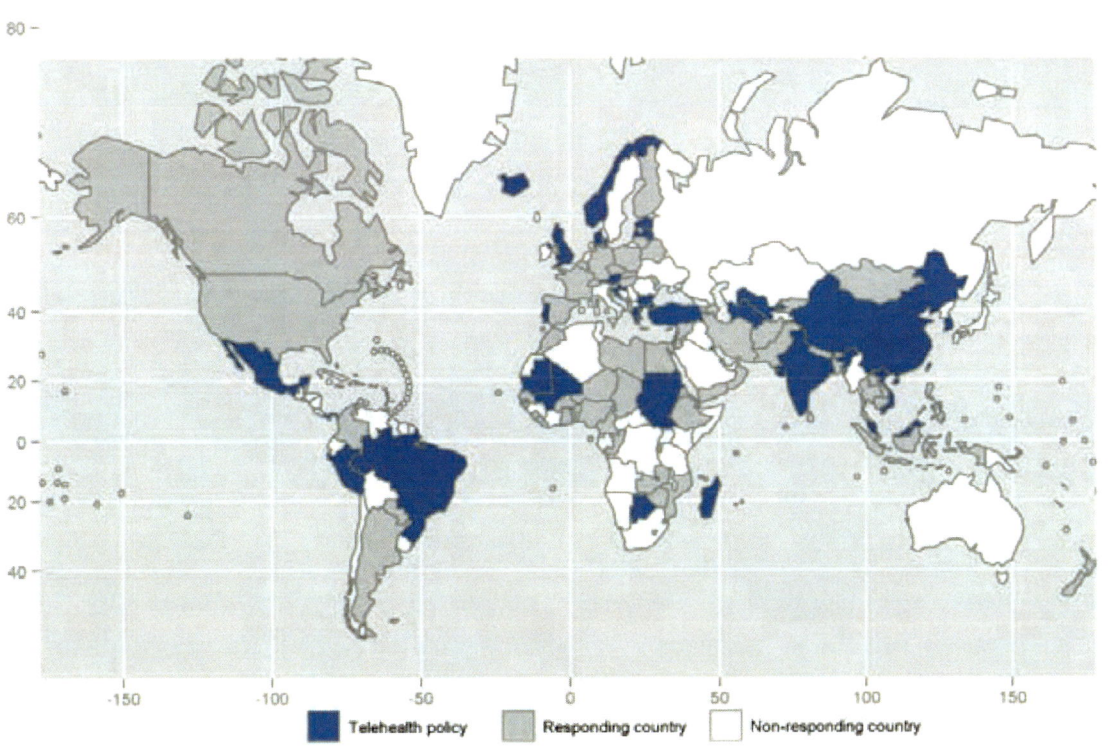

Figure 17 shows the proportion of responding countries with national telemedicine policies by WHO region. While the trends seen are similar to those seen in the establishment of telemedicine agencies, the differences between regions is more pronounced. The European Region was most advanced in this area, with approximately 40% of responding countries having a national telemedicine policy. By comparison, only 10% to 15% of responding countries in the Eastern Mediterranean, South-East Asian, and African Regions reported having such a policy.

Figure 18 shows country responses by World Bank income group. These results reflect a common trend, with high- and upper-middle income countries more likely to have such a policy than those in the lower-middle and low-income groups.

Figure 17. National telemedicine policies by WHO region

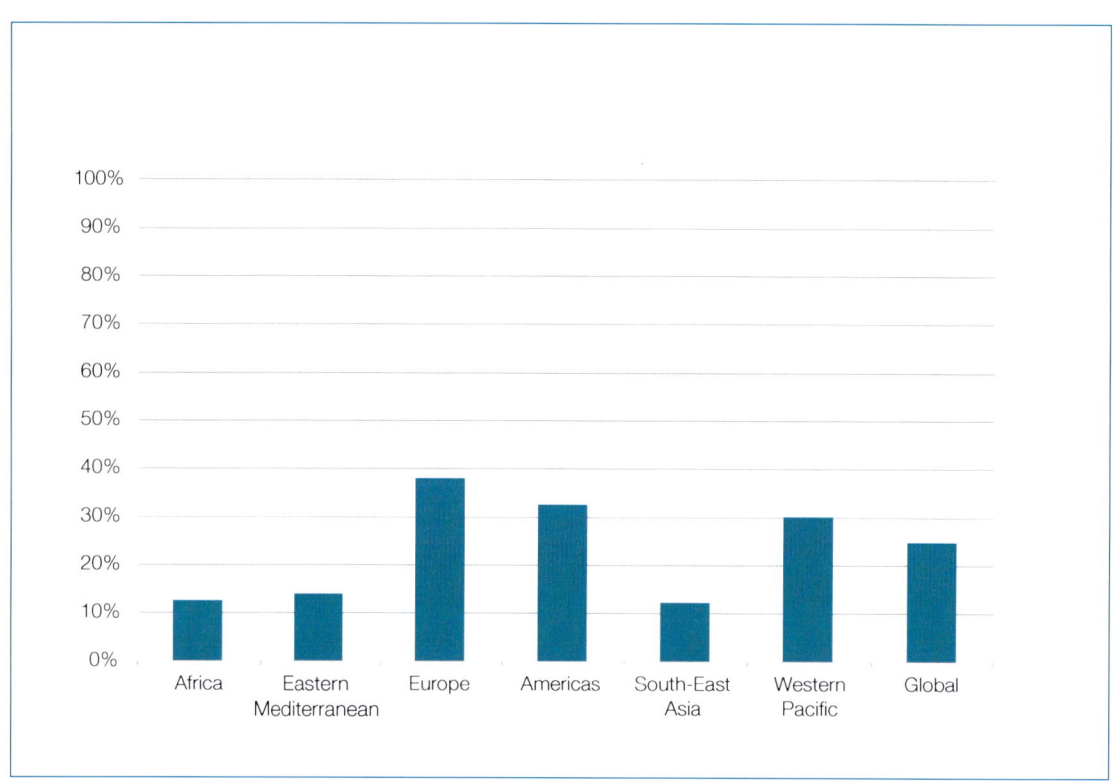

Figure 18. National telemedicine policies by World Bank income group

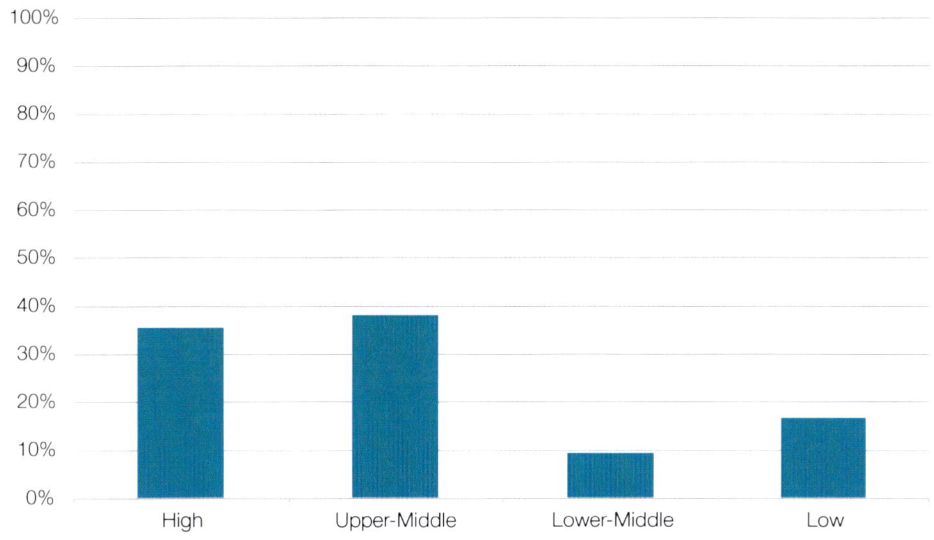

Survey respondents were also asked to report if their telemedicine policy had been implemented, and if not, when action was expected to be taken. Just over 5% of all responding countries reported that their national telemedicine policy had been fully implemented, while just over 10% reported having partially implemented their policy. A further 5% of countries stated that although they currently had a telemedicine policy, at the time of the survey no action towards implementing it had been taken.

There is a significant degree of variation between WHO regions in terms of telemedicine policy implementation. Across the Regions of the Americas, Europe and the Western Pacific, approximately 30% of responding countries reported full or partial implementation of a policy (see Figure 19). In contrast, implementation has taken place within very few countries in the Regions of Africa, the Eastern Mediterranean (both less than 10%) and South-East Asia (just over 10%). Despite this, projections given by responding countries show that by 2013, over 50% of all responding countries anticipate having developed and begun the execution of a national telemedicine policy, with an implementation rate of 45% to 75% across WHO regions. The most considerable progress in that time period is anticipated within the African, Eastern Mediterranean and South-East Asian Regions.

Figure 20 illustrates that economically developed countries are more likely to have put their national telemedicine policy into practice than developing countries. Currently, implementation has occurred in 25% to 35% of responding countries within high-income and upper-middle income groups, compared to approximately 10% of responding countries in lower-middle and low-income groups. With that said, projections indicate the potential for a marked increase in the development and implementation of telemedicine policy throughout developing countries. By 2013, it is possible that implementation rates could range from 40% to 55% across all income groups.

Figure 19. Policy implementation by WHO region

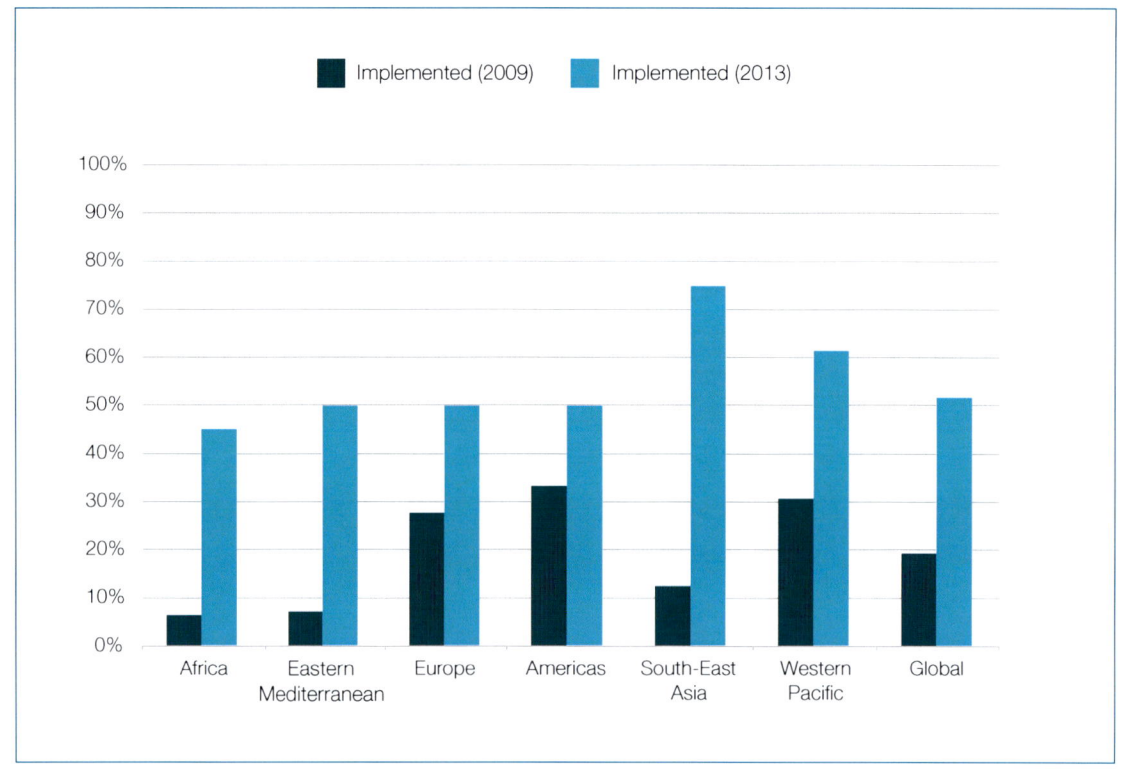

Figure 20. Policy implementation by World Bank income group

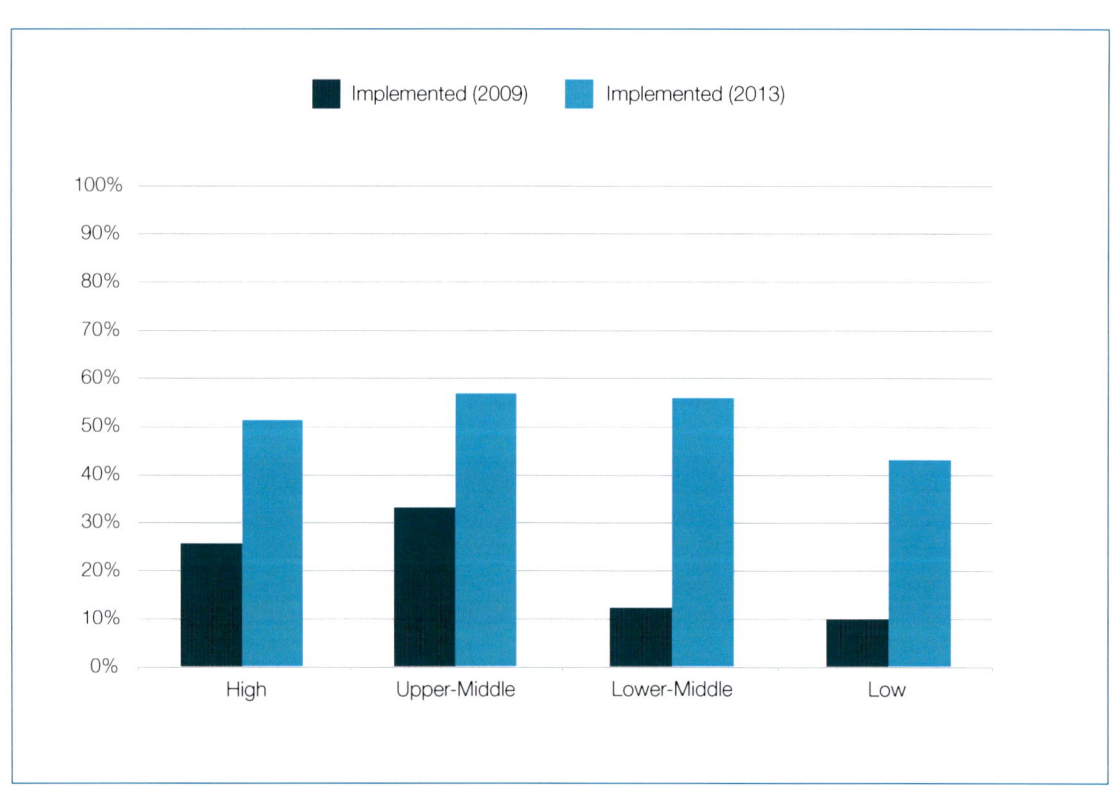

## Implications for policy and strategy

Comprehensive telemedicine policies and strategies can help support the development and adoption of telemedicine solutions, address relevant legal and ethical issues, and provide long-term benefits to health care systems. Only a small proportion of countries have developed and implemented a national telemedicine policy, and only half of the countries without a current policy are projected to have one by 2013. This mirrors the finding within the literature that definitive and comprehensive telemedicine guidelines have yet to be put into broad-based practice, and is not surprising when one considers that eHealth policies in general are less common than broader health and information policies. The lack of telemedicine policies shows that in the majority of countries there is insufficient impetus to compel policy-makers to set such policies. This may reflect a need for more evidence on the benefits of telemedicine, or a perception that benefits are insufficient to justify forming policy; it could also be due to a lack of demand from citizens or health-care professionals.

While the issue is particularly evident in developing countries, the increase in policy development projected to 2013 in the African, Eastern Mediterranean and South-East Asian Regions provides some encouragement. This reflects a potential recognition among governments and policy-makers of the benefits such policies offer in the implementation and development of telemedicine. In addition, it may signify that these countries could experience an increase in the demand and capacity for telemedicine in the future, thus assisting policy-makers to anticipate future needs in human resources for telemedicine implementation.

While the data show few countries currently have telemedicine policies, this could represent a potential opportunity: health authorities could integrate telemedicine into national health and eHealth strategies from the outset. Collaboration between policy-makers, health professionals, and citizens would greatly enhance the planning, development, and assessment of telemedicine services.

### KEY POINTS

- Half of responding countries reported that scientific institutions are currently involved in developing telemedicine solutions in their country.

- Low-income countries are just as likely to have a scientific institution engaged in the development of telemedicine solutions as high-income countries; there appears to be some collaboration between scientific institutions in high-income and low-income countries to develop and implement telemedicine solutions in low-income countries.

- The African Region has the second-highest rate of scientific institutional involvement in telemedicine development, while the Eastern Mediterranean Region has the lowest reported rate of involvement.

- In many countries scientific institutions are involved in developing telemedicine solutions in the absence of national telemedicine agencies or policies.

### 4.2.3 Scientific development

The involvement of scientific institutions in the development of telemedicine brings with it a number of potential benefits. Such institutions can dedicate resources to the development and testing of a variety of telemedicine initiatives, and ensure that telemedicine is put into practice and evaluated in a systematic manner. Institutions such as teaching hospitals can be involved in the education of the next generation of health professionals. The involvement of scientific institutions can also increase the likelihood that telemedicine innovation and implementation is documented and disseminated to others wishing to advance its development and use.

Survey respondents were asked if scientific institutions in their country are currently involved in the development of telemedicine solutions, to which 50% of countries responded in the affirmative. When asked to provide the most active institutions involved in the development of telemedicine, a broad variety of responses were provided. Institutions included government health and technology agencies, universities (primarily faculties of health or medicine), hospitals (primarily those with close ties to universities), professional societies related to eHealth and telemedicine, and dedicated research institutions with a focus on technology, communications, and health.

In five of the six regions, between 40% and 70% of responding countries have scientific institutions involved in telemedicine development; the exception to this is the Eastern Mediterranean Region, where less than 20% of countries currently report having institutional involvement (Figure 21). The involvement of scientific institutions in telemedicine development within the African Region is slightly above the global mean; the Region has the second-highest rate of institutional involvement, behind the European Region.

Figure 22 reveals an interesting result when the results are stratified by World Bank income group; the difference between income groups is not particularly large, and both high-income and low-income countries have a similar proportion of countries with scientific institutions involved in telemedicine development.

Figure 21. Institutional involvement by WHO region

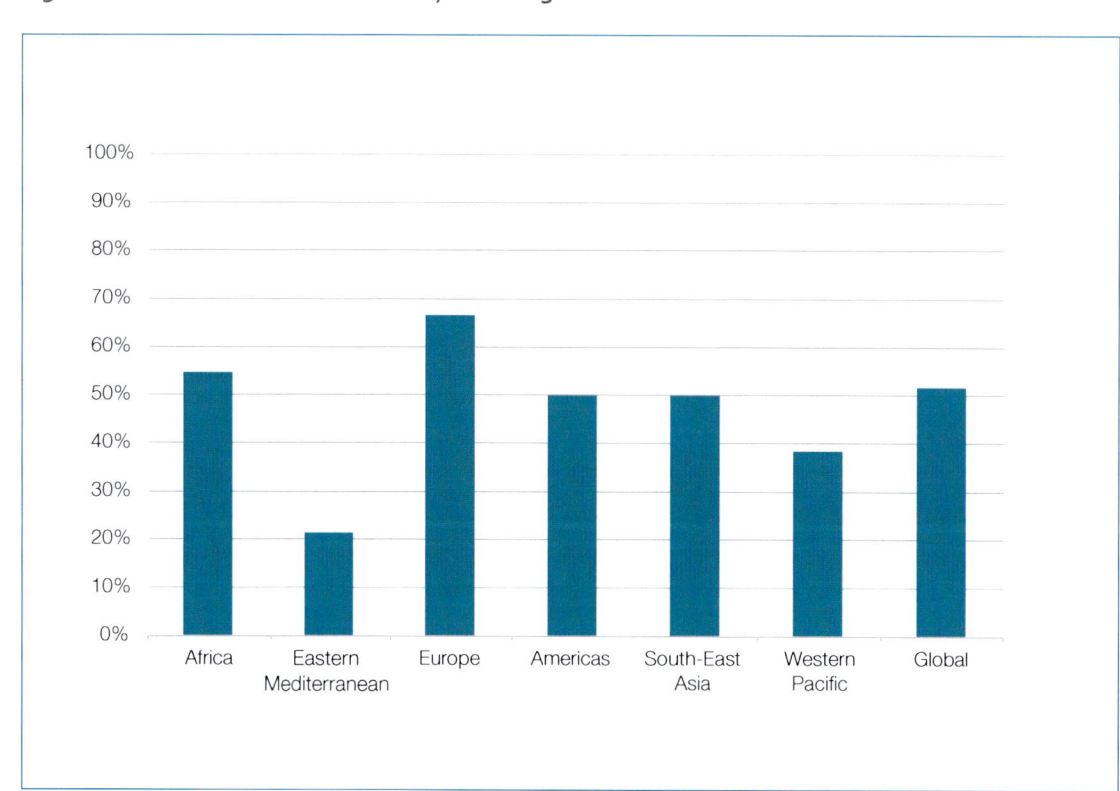

Figure 22. Institutional involvement by World Bank income group

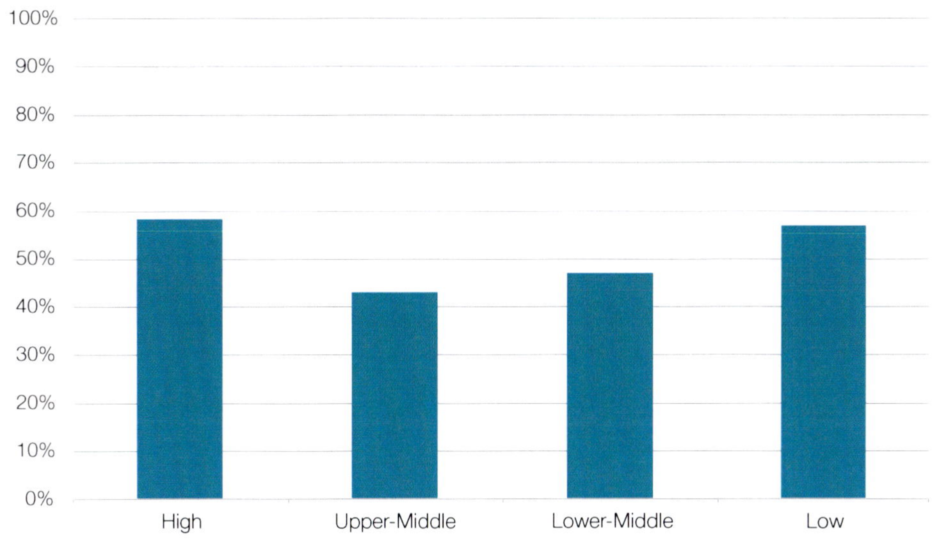

## Implications for scientific development of telemedicine

The relatively high proportion of developing countries that engage scientific institutions is encouraging. One potential benefit of their involvement in telemedicine implementation is that it provides a marker that these programmes will eventually be evaluated and documented. As such, this trend provides encouragement that future publications documenting and analysing telemedicine services, particularly those in developing countries, can be anticipated.

The data in Figure 22 could reflect increasing collaborations between high- and low-income countries to assist in the development of telemedicine solutions. The African Region, with the second-highest rate of institutional involvement, appears to show a particular interest in the use of telemedicine (Figure 21). As an example, one of the more well-established collaborative initiatives between high- and low-income countries is the RAFT Project[8] (Réseau en Afrique Francophone pour la Télémédicine). Coordinated primarily by the Geneva University Hospital in Switzerland and university hospitals in Africa, the RAFT network is active in 15 francophone African countries and focuses on telemedicine and distance education of health-care professionals working in remote sites.

- There are also factors beyond level of economic development that may influence the degree of involvement of scientific institutions in the development of telemedicine.
- Countries may recognize the need to properly develop and evaluate telemedicine applications.
- Availability of funding, either locally or internationally, may attract scientific institutions to apply for, and participate in research and development.
- Countries may engage scientific institutions to participate in conducting cross-country comparisons of telemedicine applications to stimulate knowledge exchange.
- Members of scientific institutions (faculty members or students) may desire to undertake fieldwork for both research and service learning.

8  http://raft.hcuge.ch/ and http://www.comminit.com/en/node/126900/307.

Based on the survey results, it would be informative to further explore the various factors leading to the engagement of scientific institutions, and to monitor the relationship between institutional involvement and the production of scientific publications, both in terms of quantity and quality.

Another point of interest would be to investigate the types of international collaborations taking place between scientific institutions and foreign countries, and explore how these projects evolve from being externally to internally funded, and achieve long-term sustainability. Furthermore, it would be worthwhile to examine in more detail the direction of engagement between high- and low-income countries. Determining which countries instigate contact for collaborative purposes would provide further insight into the degree of assistance high-income countries are willing and able to offer for telemedicine development in developing countries, as well as the type and degree of expertise requested by low-income countries.

One further noteworthy observation is that the proportion of countries with institutions involved in telemedicine development is considerably greater than the proportion of countries with national telemedicine agencies or policies, particularly within the African Region. This suggests that many institutions are developing telemedicine solutions in the absence of policies or governance in place at the national level. It would be of particular interest to follow the relationship between these two factors. This will help determine how the development of telemedicine is influenced by the presence of a national telemedicine policy, and how the development and entrenchment of telemedicine policy occurs in countries where scientific institutions are involved with the development of telemedicine solutions and evidence.

> **KEY POINTS**
> - Only 20% of responding countries reported having evaluated or reviewed the use of telemedicine in their country since 2006.
> - Low-income countries are almost as likely as high-income countries to have an evaluation of telemedicine use in their country published recently.
> - The African, Eastern Mediterranean and Western Pacific Regions all have a smaller proportion of countries with recently-published evaluations of telemedicine use than the proportion found worldwide.

### 4.2.4 Evaluation processes

Rigorous evaluation processes play a vital role in the progress of any medical field, and telemedicine is no different. Conducting evaluations and disseminating results may be particularly important to the field of telemedicine given the scarcity of empirical evidence on its use. These evaluations can help generate reliable data to develop national telemedicine policy and strategy, streamline telemedicine implementation, and inform the potential for enhancement and transferability of telemedicine projects. The following case study highlights an example of a programme that has evaluated its success and impact throughout the course of its existence.

# The Swinfen Charitable Trust Telemedicine Network

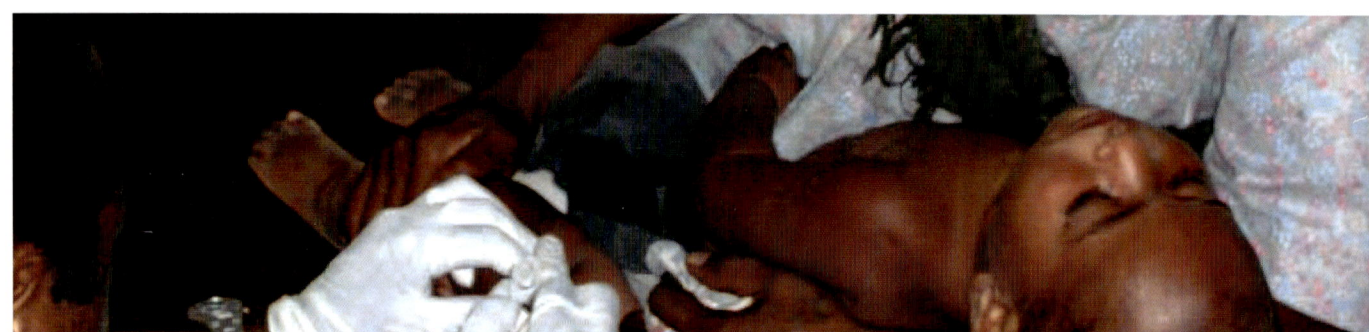

The Swinfen Charitable Trust Telemedicine Network uses a low-cost, store-and-forward telemedicine system to link health-care workers in developing countries to an international pool of consulting specialists. Based in the United Kingdom, the network is operated by the Swinfen Charitable Trust (SCT), a completely volunteer organization.

Since the first telemedicine link in 1999, the network has grown to include 193 referring hospitals and clinics from over 60 counties. At inception the network was based on a simple e-mailing system between the referring health-care professionals and the consulting physicians. The method of communication has been enhanced to a Web-based messaging system that only requires an Internet connection and no special software. All involved parties are able to log into one private and secure centralized system. The details of the clinical case, including images such as clinical photographs or X-rays, are posted on the message board with a request for advice from specialists from one or more areas of expertise.

Submission of the referral to the message board prompts an e-mail to the SCT to inform the recipient that a new referral has been posted. After the SCT system operators review the referral they send an e-mail to the appropriate volunteer specialist. Once notified of the referral via an e-mail prompt the appointed specialist logs onto the message board to review the clinical information, and respond to the referral. In addition to accessing the details of the clinical case, the specialist can view information about the hospital or clinic from where the referral is generated in order to determine the scope of available diagnostic tests and services.

The Swinfen Charitable Trust Network receives approximately 250 referrals per year, and the average time between the initial posting by the referring health-care worker and the first response by a consulting physician is approximately 19–24 hours.

The service is of particular benefit to physicians who work in remote regions with limited access to diagnostic testing, as without this service they would not have access to a second opinion and advice from specialists with expertise in such a range of clinical areas. The network has also benefitted patients and their families, especially those who are not able to travel long distances to obtain specialty health care services.

Various aspects of the network's services have been documented including user satisfaction, speed of response to referral, quality of clinical images, and the role of medical students to facilitate the use of the service by physicians working in hospitals who are linked to the network.[1,2,3,4] Overall, referring physicians consider the advice from the specialists to be helpful, particularly in establishing a diagnosis, and providing reassurance to the health care team, patient, and the patient's family.[3] Academic papers reporting on the work of the SCT can be obtained from the Trust's website at: www.swinfencharitabletrust.org.

To evolve existing methods of service provision, the SCT hopes to further integrate the exchange of information via mobile phones with high-resolution cameras. Using hand-held devices can expedite the consultation process by increasing accessibility from where a referral is submitted. The SCT would also like to respond to increasing requests for services in multiple languages. Currently, the SCT is in the trial phase of a system in both English and French with Médecins Sans Frontières. The SCT is also working with a Greek Medical Charity to set up a system in Greek to support a hospital that serves a Greek community in the United Republic of Tanzania, and there are plans to set up a system in Spanish for doctors in Bolivia.

Acknowledgements
Lord and Lady Swinfen,
Founders and Directors, Swinfen Charitable Trust

### References

1. Jakowenko J, Wootton R. An analysis of the images attached to referral messages in an e-mail-based telemedicine system for developing countries. *Journal of Telemedicine and Telecare*, 2006, 12(Suppl. 3):S49–S53.
2. Patterson V et al. Supporting hospital doctors in the Middle East by e-mail telemedicine. *Journal of Medical Internet Research*, 2007, 9(4):e30.
3. Wootton R, Menzies J, Ferguson P. Follow-up data for patients managed by store and forward telemedicine in developing countries. *Journal of Telemedicine and Telecare*, 2009, 15(2):83–88.
4. Wootton R et al. Medical students represent a valuable resource in facilitating telehealth for the under-served. Journal of Telemedicine and Telecare, 2007, 13(Suppl. 3):S3.

Respondents were asked about the level of evaluation and review that has taken place with regards to telemedicine service use, in particular the publication of recent evaluation reports or review studies on the use of telemedicine services in their country. For the purpose of this report, the terms 'evaluation' and 'review' are used interchangeably. Only 20% of countries reported having published an evaluation report or review study on the use of telemedicine in their country published since 2006. The content of the evaluations and reviews submitted by responding countries varied somewhat in their content and methodology; less than half of these evaluations were specific, methodologically-sound evaluations of telemedicine, with the majority being more general overview documents on the use of telemedicine or other eHealth initiatives within the country. It seems that detailed, high-quality evaluations of telemedicine, incorporating detailed results such as patient outcomes or cost–benefit analyses, are being conducted and disseminated by very few countries.

Figure 23 depicts the results by WHO region. While the European Region has the highest proportion of countries with a recently published evaluation of telemedicine use (just under 30%), there is not a great deal of difference between regions; the lowest proportion was 15% in the Eastern Mediterranean Region. In most regions, the proportion of countries with a recently published evaluation was approximately half the proportion of those with scientific institutions involved with telemedicine development. In the African Region, the proportion of countries with recently published evaluations (just over 15%) was less than a third of those with scientific institutions involved in developing telemedicine (55%).

Figure 24 shows another trend of interest with regard to country income. While the difference between income groups is not large, both high- and low-income groups have a similar proportion of countries that have recently published an evaluation or review of telemedicine. This trend parallels that seen in Figure 22; given academic institutions and donors in high-income countries often target low-income countries for telemedicine programmes, the trend is not unusual. These programmes often would be evaluated for academic publication, or assessed internally by the donor organization.

Figure 23. Published evaluation by WHO region

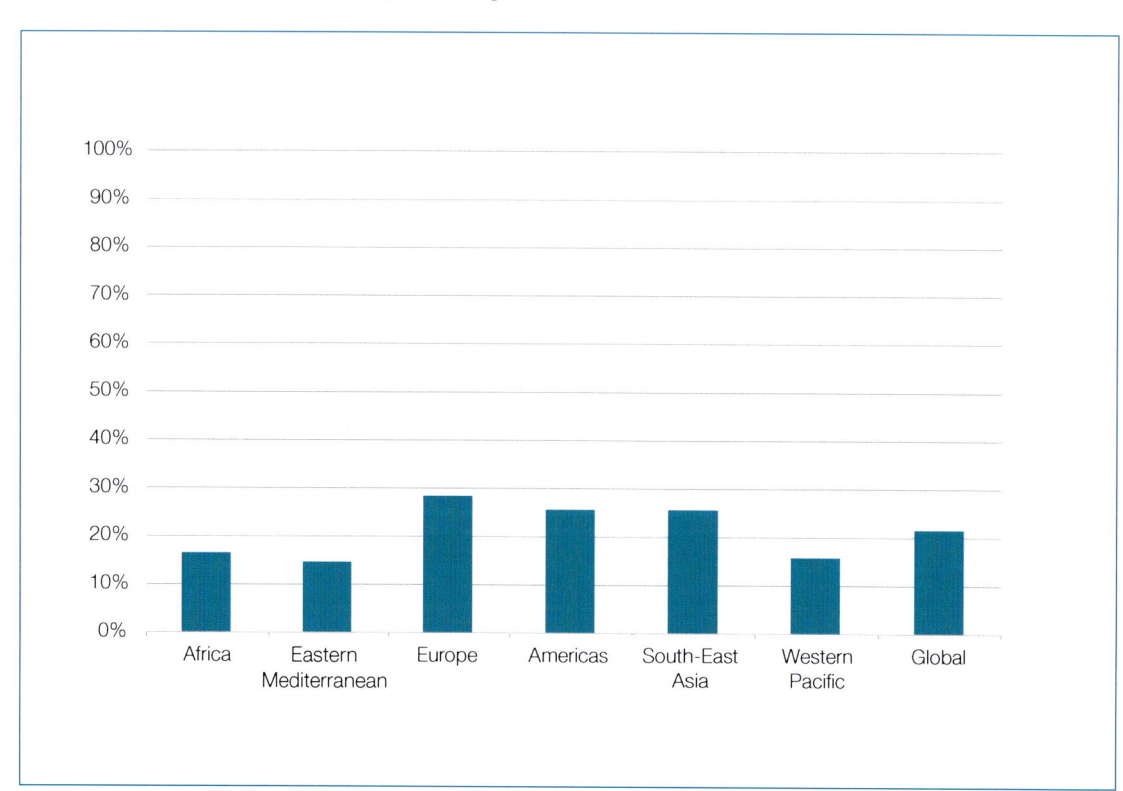

Figure 24. Published evaluation by World Bank income group

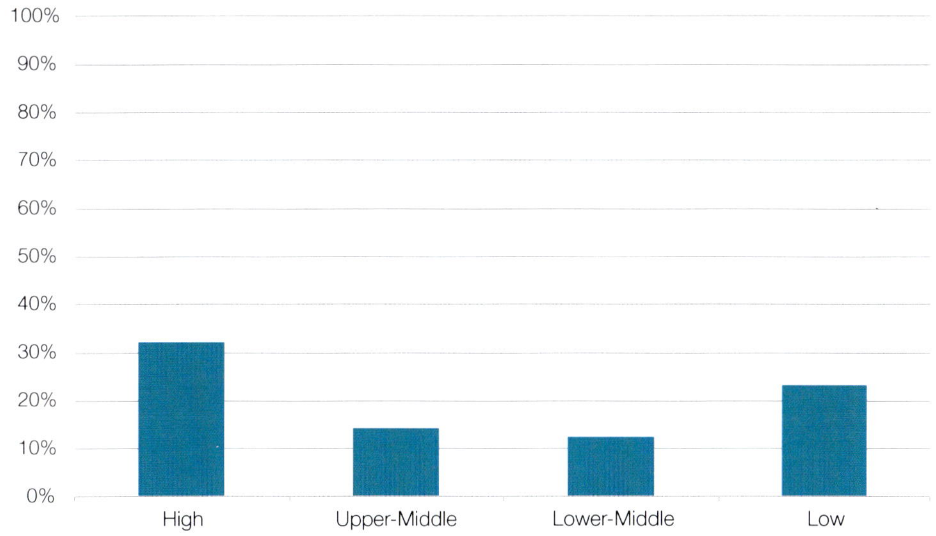

## Implications for evaluation processes in telemedicine

Rigorous evaluations of telemedicine initiatives are required to generate reliable data for use by policy-makers to create and shape national telemedicine policy and strategies. Best practices, lessons learnt, and economic and health outcomes should be documented and published by institutions developing telemedicine solutions; this can provide models that help streamline implementation processes, inform the modification of existing projects for cost-effectiveness and scalability, and assess the transferability of initiatives across locations and medical specialty. While careful planning and evaluation of telemedicine initiatives is always important, these processes become a key component of helping to ensure limited resources are utilized in an optimal manner.

It is interesting to note the similar trend shown between country income and published evaluation, and income and institutional involvement in telemedicine research, with the highest participation found among countries with the highest and lowest income incomes. The survey did not ask respondents whether their evaluation was published by local authorities or international collaborators; the results may further reflect partnerships between high- and low-income countries, and a desire in high-income countries to evaluate and publish on the development and effectiveness of telemedicine solutions in low-income countries. However, the disparity found in the African Region between the high proportion of countries with scientific institutions involved in telemedicine and the low proportion of countries with published evaluations of telemedicine services does raise questions as to why evaluation was not more common in the region.

The survey results suggest there is a paucity of published telemedicine evaluation and trial data results, not only in developing countries, but also globally. Only one in five responding countries had a formal telemedicine evaluation recently published, less than half the proportion of countries with scientific institutions involved with developing telemedicine solutions. Possible explanations for this discrepancy between institutional involvement and the publication of evaluations are many and varied, but may include:

- lack of research expertise or funding to support evaluation;
- bias towards spending funding on implementation of telemedicine solutions rather than research and evaluation;
- difficulty in obtaining a sufficient sample of patients for evaluation;
- bias towards only publishing evaluations of successful projects;
- the time required for a programme to become established and considered successful; and
- long periods between project completion, article writing, and eventual publication.

There may well be other factors present or other distinct obstacles affecting the low rate of evaluation. It would be interesting to further explore and validate the various reasons for this relative lack of evaluation and address them, which may raise evaluation activities and contribute to future evidence-informed telemedicine development.

Many of the barriers listed above are exacerbated when telemedicine services are informal in nature. For example, it may be impossible to find a suitable patient sample or obtain follow-up data for telemedicine services that are not part of a formal programme, or where populations are widely dispersed and remote. The relatively short lifespan of most telemedicine initiatives, especially if informal in nature, reduces the chances of the initiative becoming established, or formal evaluations and reviews being performed and published. The relatively high proportion of informal services reported in the Eastern Mediterranean, African and Western Pacific Regions have likely had a large bearing on explaining the relatively low proportion of countries with recently published evidence in these regions. It is clear that further assistance to conduct and publish telemedicine research and evaluation is likely required in each of these regions.

The current lack of research and evaluation has the potential to undermine the development of telemedicine services, and threaten support for its future implementation. Of concern is the possibility that telemedicine implementation is occurring without formal evaluation or review processes; these mechanisms play a vital role in determining the effectiveness and efficiency of telemedicine initiatives, and their further development vis-à-vis the most appropriate use of available resources. If evaluations are conducted but their findings are not published or disseminated, then valuable knowledge and information on telemedicine may be lost.

## 4.3 Barriers to telemedicine

### KEY POINTS

- The most prevalent barrier to the implementation of telemedicine programmes globally is the perception that costs of telemedicine are too high.

- Developing countries are more likely to consider resource issues such as high costs, underdeveloped infrastructure, and lack of technical expertise to be barriers to telemedicine.

- Developed countries are more likely to consider legal issues surrounding patient privacy and confidentiality, competing health system priorities, and a perceived lack of demand to be barriers to telemedicine implementation.

To examine the potential barriers facing countries in their implementation of telemedicine services, survey respondents were asked to select, from a list of ten potential barriers, the four that most particularly applied to their country's situation. While this type of force-choice question could potentially bias results, it was used in this large survey as a method to standardize the responses. Figure 25 shows that on a global level, by far the most prevalent reported barrier was the perceived high costs involved, with 60% of responding countries considering this a barrier to the implementation of telemedicine solutions. No other issue was as widely reported to have a negative impact on telemedicine implementation.

Figure 25. Barriers to telemedicine globally

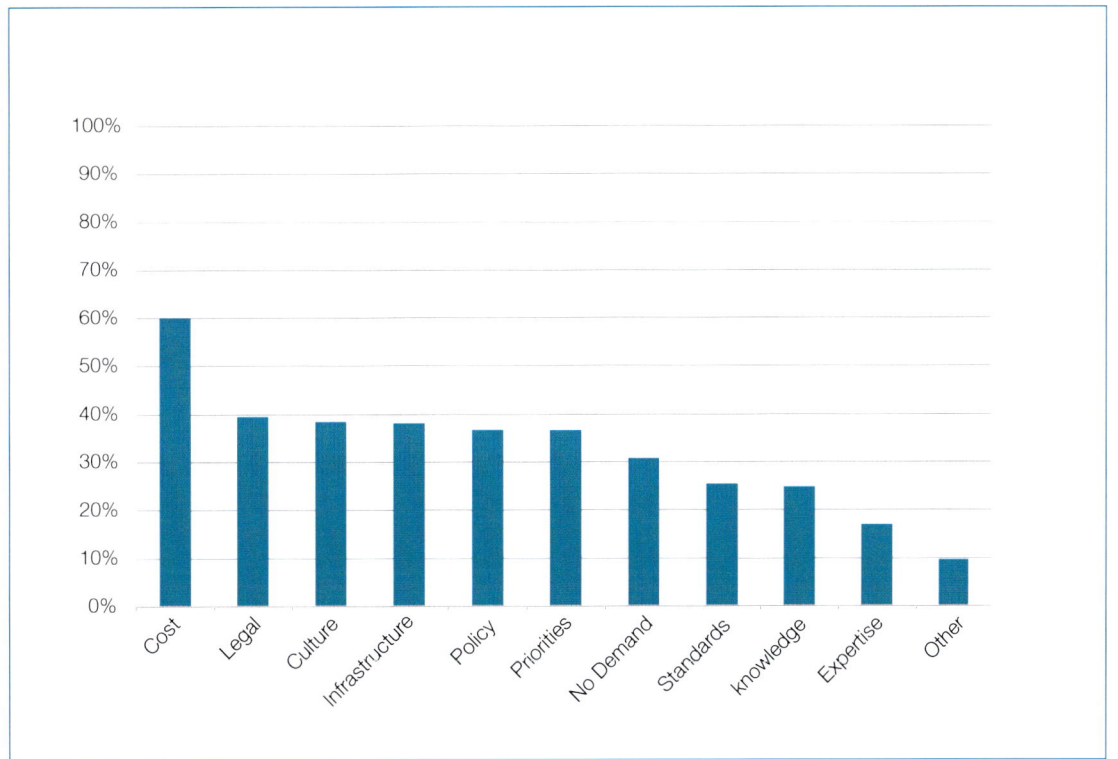

The four most prevalent barriers reported within each WHO region, alongside the global prevalence rate of that barrier, are illustrated in Figures 26 through 31; each region is displayed separately to illustrate the most significant impediments faced within each.

The perceived cost of telemedicine was among the four most commonly reported barriers to implementation in all six WHO regions, with over 50% countries in each region reporting this to be a barrier; in four of the six regions it was the most commonly reported barrier. The European and Eastern Mediterranean Regions were the only exceptions, and were the only two regions where the proportion of countries reporting cost to be a barrier was less than the global proportion. Countries in the Regions of Africa, the Americas, and South-East Asia frequently cited underdeveloped infrastructure as a barrier. The results seem to indicate that these three regions were most affected by cost and infrastructure barriers, with more countries in these regions regarding them as barriers than the level reported globally. While not necessarily indicative of a lack of physical resources, a considerable proportion of countries in the Regions of the Eastern Mediterranean and the Western Pacific reported that other issues within their health systems took priority over telemedicine and acted as a barrier to implementation.

The presence of organizational cultures unaccustomed to sharing skills and knowledge with remote professionals and patients through ICTs was found to be an important barrier in four WHO regions. Similarly, not having a national health policy or strategy that includes telemedicine as a potential approach for addressing health-related issues was found to be a considerable barrier in four WHO regions, the exceptions being the Regions of Europe and the Americas. While a lack of legal policies or guidelines on the privacy of patient information in telemedicine was the second-most commonly reported barrier on a global level, only three regions listed it among their most prevalent issues. Its high global prevalence appears primarily due to a disproportionately high percentage of countries in the European Region (close to 60%) that considered this to be a barrier.

Figure 26. Barriers for the African Region

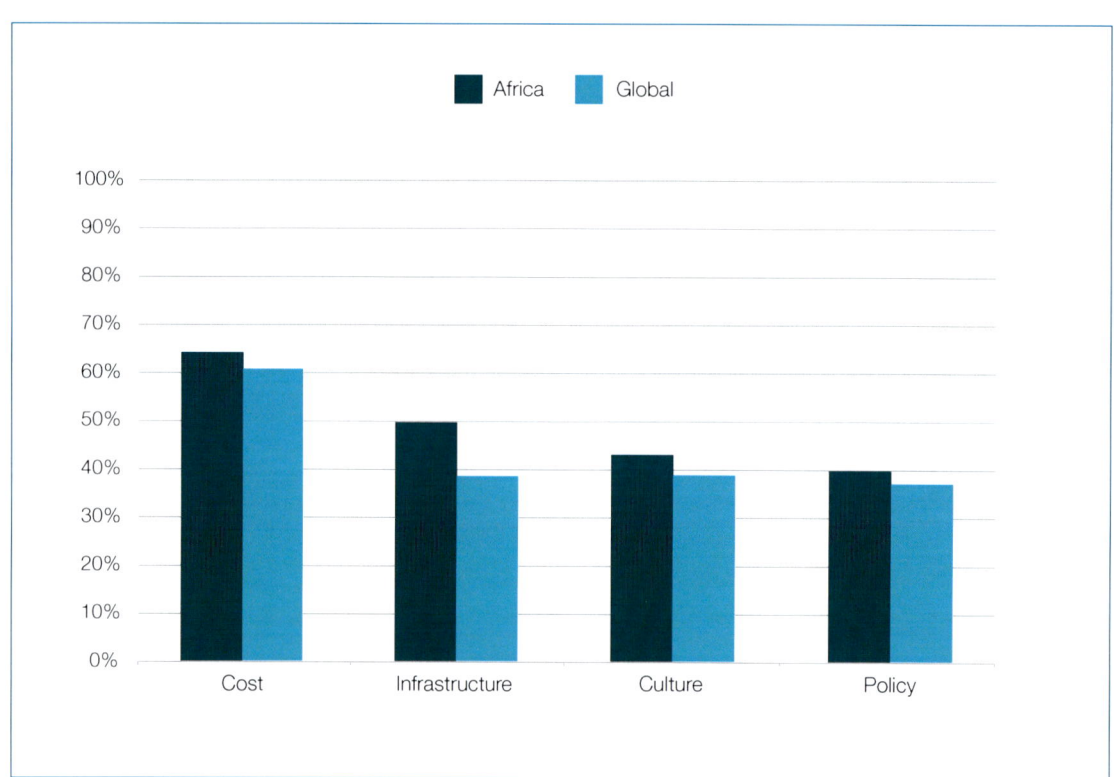

Figure 27. Barriers for the Eastern Mediterranean Region

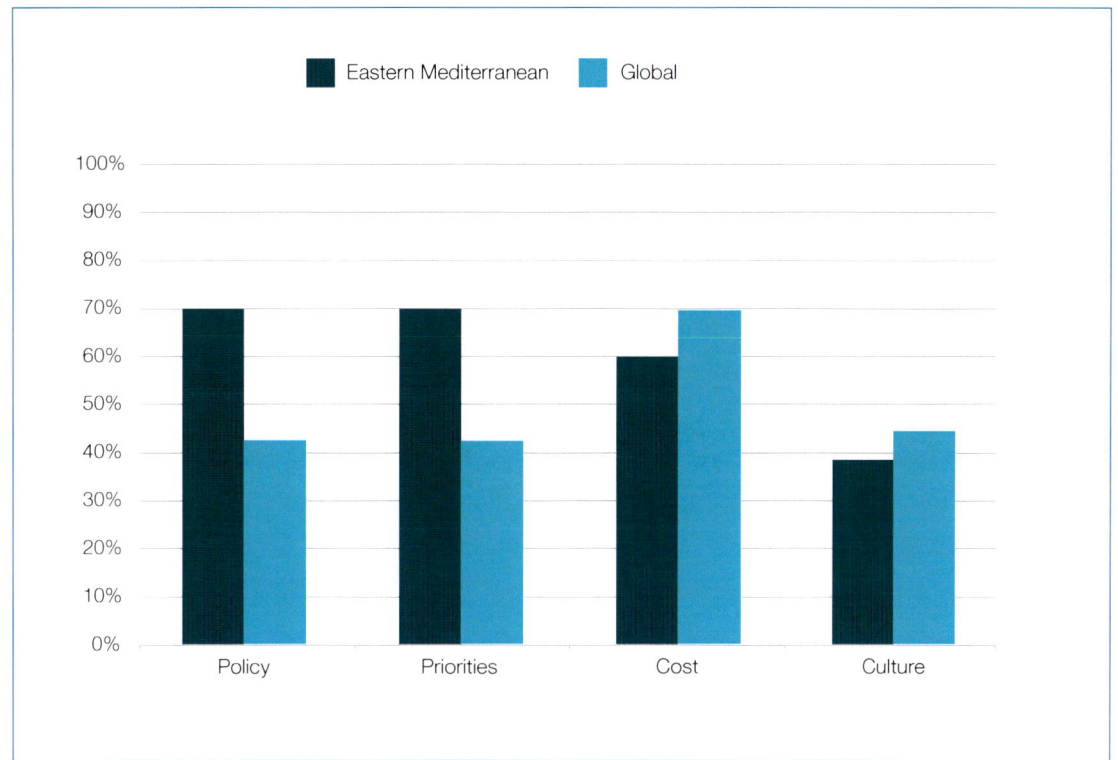

Figure 28. Barriers for the European Region

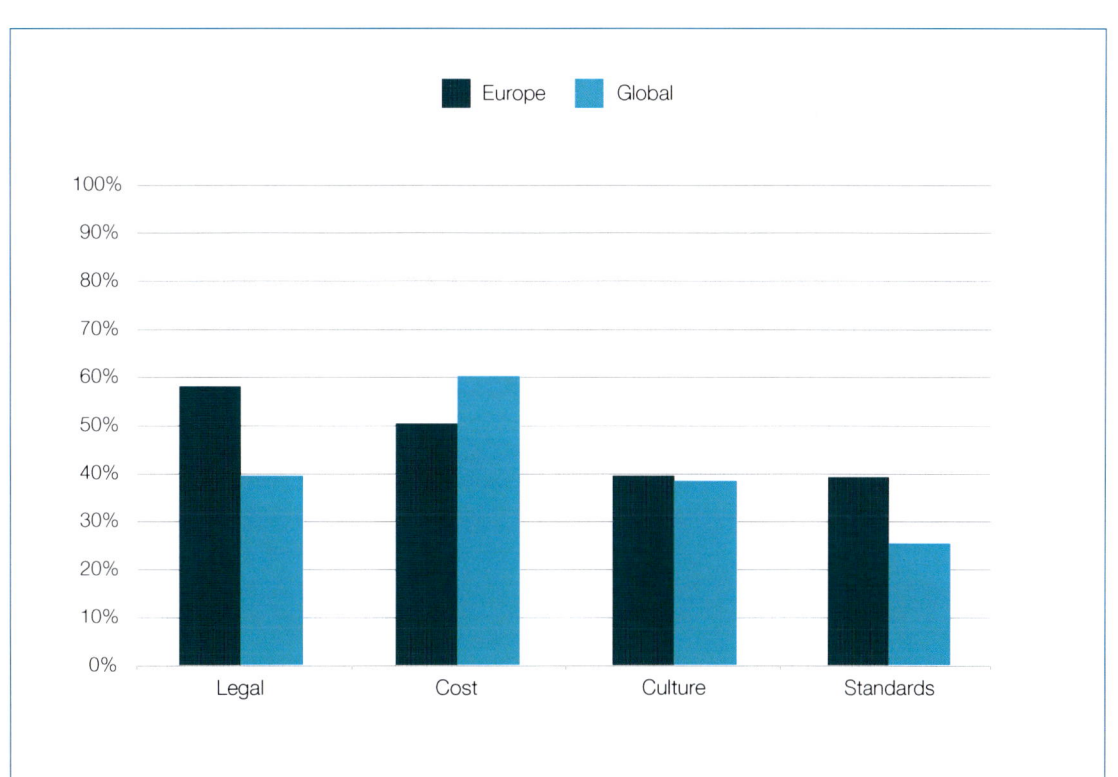

Figure 29. Barriers for the Region of the Americas

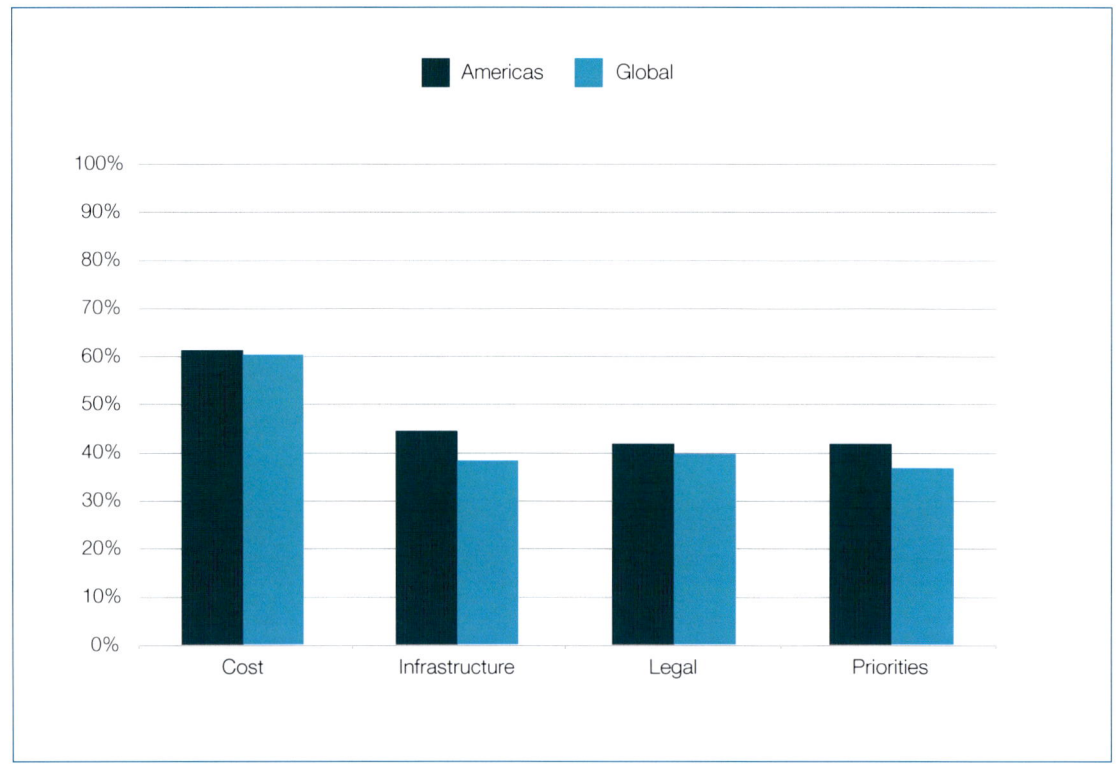

Figure 30. Barriers for the South-East Asia Region

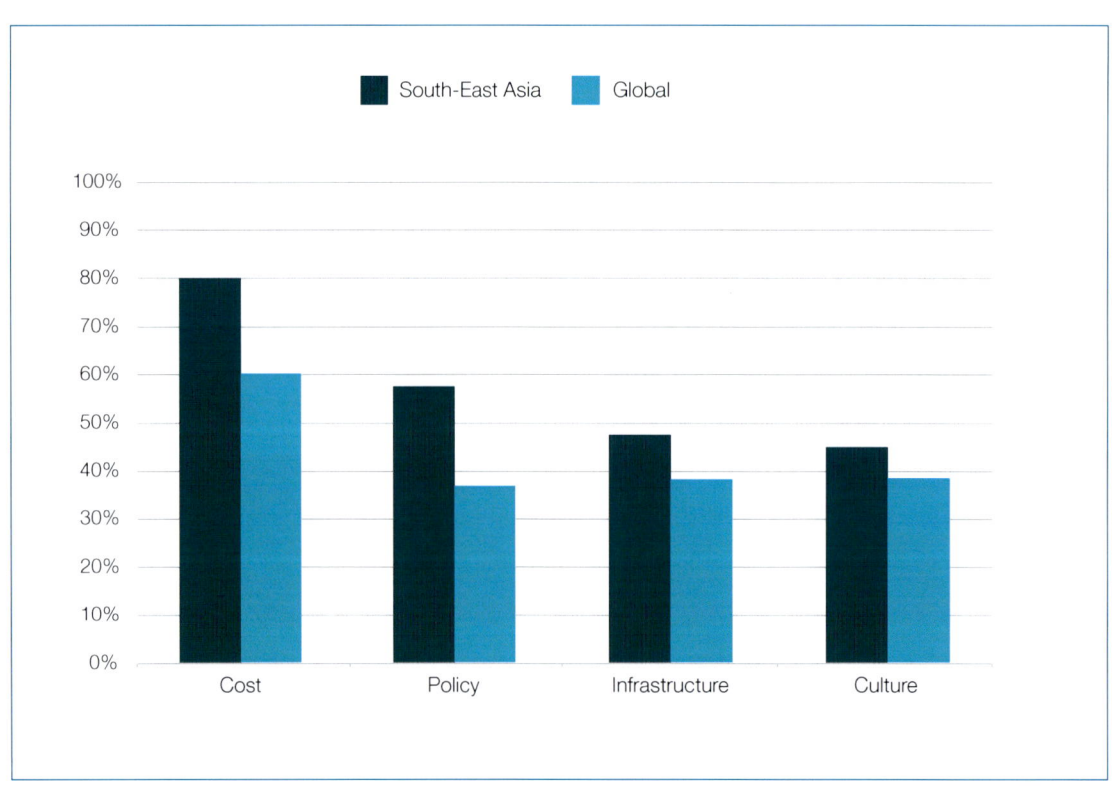

Figure 31. Barriers for the Western Pacific Region

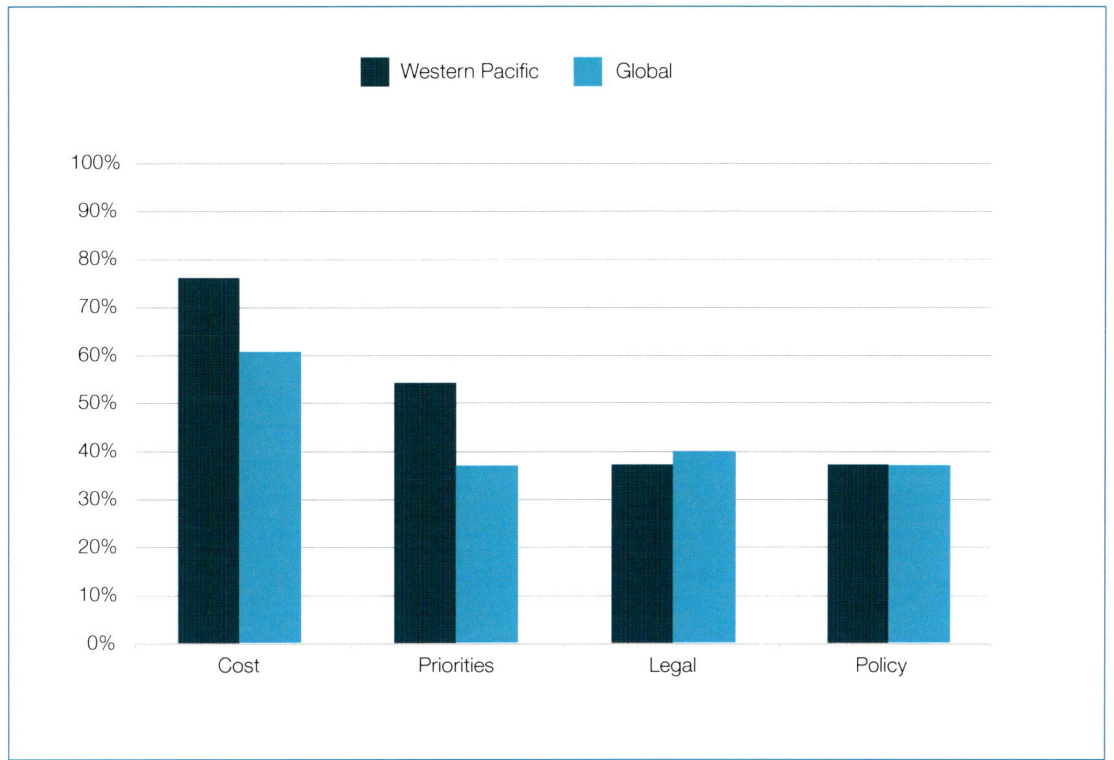

Figure 32 shows the barriers to telemedicine classified by World Bank income group. To better illustrate trends between barriers and country income levels, all ten barriers from the survey have been presented in descending order by global prevalence.

The results reveal a number of trends in differences between higher- and lower-income countries. With regards to resource issues, low- and lower-middle income countries were generally more likely to consider the perceived high costs of telemedicine solutions, an underdeveloped infrastructure, and a lack of technical expertise and support for telemedicine systems to be barriers to its implementation than developed countries. They were also more likely than upper-middle and high-income countries to report that not having a national policy or strategy that includes telemedicine solutions as a viable solution to health issues is a barrier to implementation. Low-income countries were more likely to identify a lack of knowledge of telemedicine applications available for patient treatment as a barrier.

In contrast, countries in the high- and upper-middle income groups were more likely to find issues such as a lack of legal policies or guidelines on privacy and confidentiality of patient information in telemedicine, competing priorities within their health systems, and a perceived lack of demand for telemedicine solutions by health professionals to be barriers to telemedicine. High-income countries were more likely than low-income countries to find a lack of nationally-adopted standards for telemedicine to be a barrier.

Figure 32. Barriers by World Bank income group

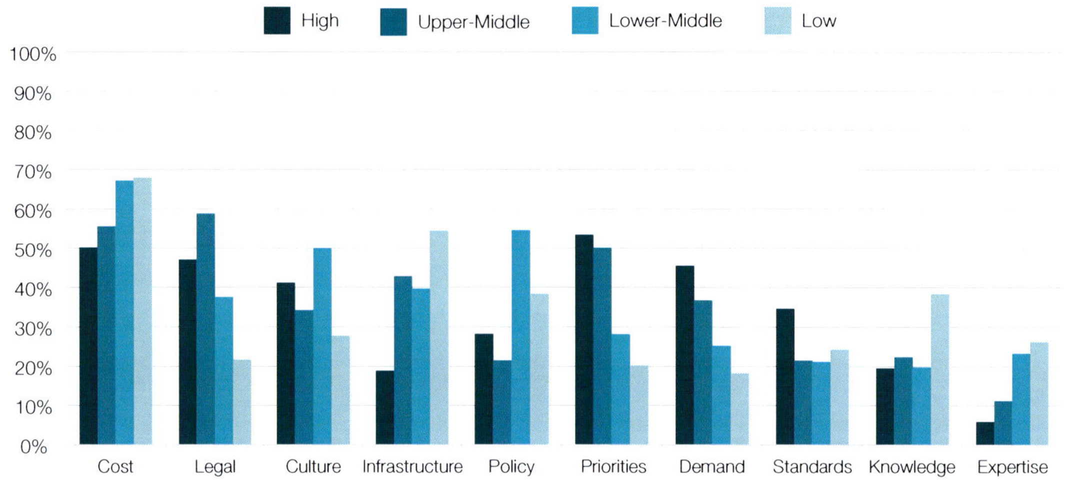

### 4.3.1 Implications for barriers to telemedicine

By far the most reported barrier to implementation of telemedicine was that the costs involved are perceived to be too high. At least half of the responding countries in each income group felt this to be a barrier, affirming that cost of equipment, maintenance, staff training, and transportation required for telemedicine is a daunting issue for governments and health providers. One possible reason for this is that telemedicine has not yet proven its value in cost-effectiveness or access and quality improvement compared to traditional health service delivery models. If there was convincing evidence to show that telemedicine programmes led to better access for patients and are more cost effective than conventional approaches, with clear economic analysis to prove the cases, cost may not have been so widely cited as an important barrier. This suggests a definite need for further evaluations of the cost–benefit of telemedicine to support its business case.

The survey results highlighting the barriers faced by developing countries – cost, underdeveloped infrastructure, and a shortage of technical expertise and support – are supported by the literature findings. Concerns regarding the implied costs of telemedicine are amplified in developing countries, particularly those with little or no funding from government or other health care organizations. Infrastructure challenges such as unstable power supplies, insufficient communication networks, and inadequate or unreliable Internet connectivity with limited bandwidth as well as a lack of human resources with the necessary technical expertise all limit where and to what degree telemedicine initiatives can be applied.

Survey results found developing countries were less likely to have a national telemedicine policy or strategy implemented; these countries were also more likely to report that lack of a national strategy or policy that includes telemedicine as an approach to health service delivery hampers its development and implementation. This finding reinforces the positive impact the presence of detailed policy and strategy frameworks can have on the development, adoption and continual assessment of telemedicine services. It also indicates that incorporating telemedicine solutions into national health policy and strategy may be of greater importance in developing countries than in developed countries, where telemedicine initiatives are frequently developed and put in place with policy and legislation on their use introduced retrospectively. While not always feasible, it is preferable – and may provide greatest benefit – to develop these structures before widespread telemedicine development and implementation commences.

Compared to lower-income countries – where access to health-care providers and the meeting of basic health needs are the first priority – developed countries generally have better infrastructure and their populations greater access to resources and health services. As such, developed countries generally have a greater number and wider array of health initiatives competing with, and potentially taking precedence over, telemedicine initiatives. In addition, legal issues surrounding patient information, privacy and confidentiality are considered to be of greater importance in telemedicine implementation. In these countries, addressing these ethical and legal issues relative to increasing health service access could yield higher uptake of telemedicine.

The third-most prevalent barrier reported globally was an organizational culture unaccustomed with the sharing and exchange of knowledge and skills with professionals and patients located in remote locations via ICT. This challenge in change management is independent of country income, available resources, or regional need for telemedicine solutions. As the adoption of telemedicine systems requires the acceptance of users involved in the process, this finding may indicate a lack of awareness of, or comfort in, the use of telemedicine systems. As a result, global and concerted advocacy on the benefits and the appropriate use of telemedicine would help address fears or resistance towards technology use and accelerate its adoption among health professionals and patients alike.

### KEY POINTS

- Resource issues were a common information requirement, with almost 70% of countries desiring further information on the cost and cost-effectiveness of telemedicine solutions, and over 50% of countries wanting more information on the infrastructure necessary to implement telemedicine solutions.

- Five of six WHO regions found that information on the cost and cost-effectiveness of telemedicine solutions was their greatest telemedicine information need.

- Further information on the clinical uses of telemedicine was required by almost 60% of responding countries, and was found to be among the three most requested areas of information in all six WHO regions.

- While differences between income groups were generally not great, high-income countries were most likely to want further information on the cost and cost-effectiveness of telemedicine, while low-income countries were more likely to require information on the infrastructure necessary for telemedicine.

## 4.4 Telemedicine information needs

To gain an understanding of the information needs surrounding telemedicine, survey respondents were asked to select, from a list of seven, the four most important areas of information that their country required to support the development of telemedicine. Figure 33 displays the information needs reported by all responding countries. Resource issues were again seen as a major point of concern, with almost 70% of responding countries desiring further information on the cost and cost-effectiveness of telemedicine solutions, while over 50% of countries wanted more information on the infrastructure necessary to implement telemedicine solutions. Information on the clinical uses of telemedicine was the second-most cited information need – by almost 60% of responding countries.

Figure 33. Information needs of all countries

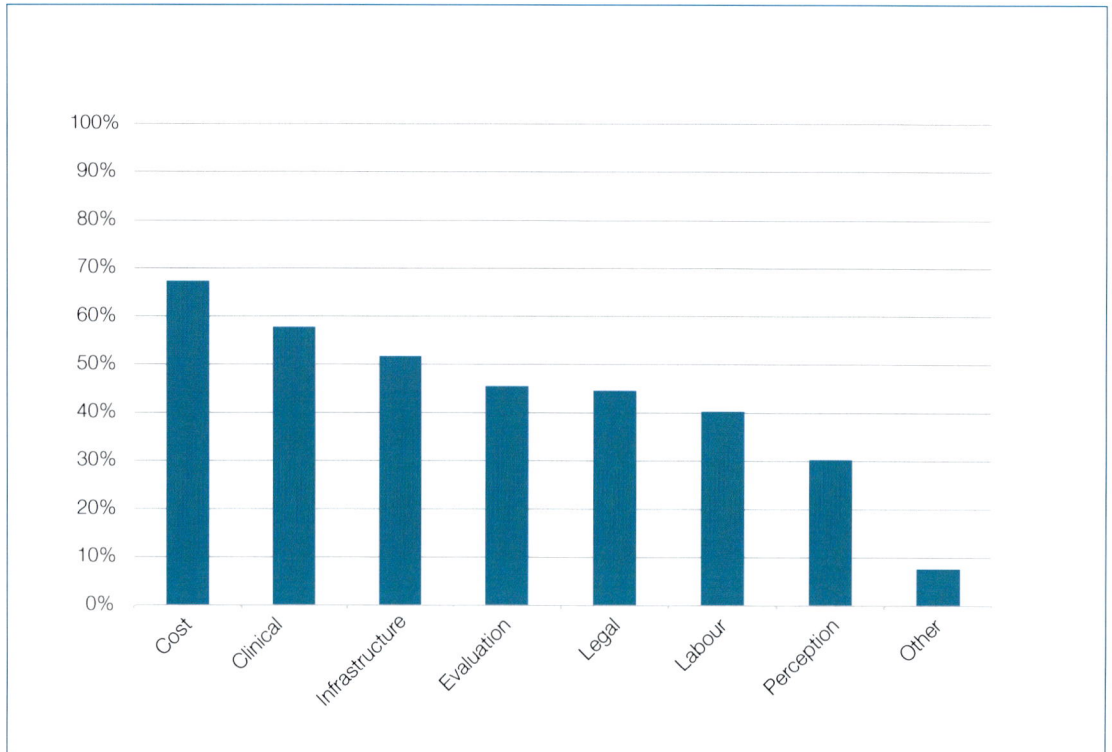

The four greatest information needs reported by each WHO region, alongside the global prevalence, are shown in Figures 34 through 39; each region is displayed separately to illustrate the unique needs of each. Results show that information needs on telemedicine appear to be generally similar between regions.

Information on the cost of telemedicine was the most pressing information need in five of the six WHO regions. Approximately 85% of countries in the Americas desired more information on this area. The Eastern Mediterranean and African Regions were the only two regions in which the proportion of countries that required information on the costs of telemedicine (40% and 60%, respectively) was lower than the global rate. It is also interesting to note that in the Eastern Mediterranean Region, approximately 75% of countries desired information on the infrastructure necessary for telemedicine implementation. This may suggest that within this region there is less concern over availability of financial resources, and a greater desire to develop and establish telemedicine infrastructure in the near future.

Information on the clinical uses of telemedicine was found to be among the three most requested areas of information in all WHO regions, showing this to be a significant need at the global level and not just in particular regions. Other information needs that countries frequently cited were the need for information on legal and ethical aspects of telemedicine, and the need for research publications evaluating the effects of telemedicine on quality of services; both of these areas were among the most commonly cited in three WHO regions. There was also a particular interest in labour issues within the Region of the Americas, with just over 60% of countries citing the need for more information on the effect of telemedicine on the use of human resources in the health care sector.

Figure 34. Information needs of the African Region

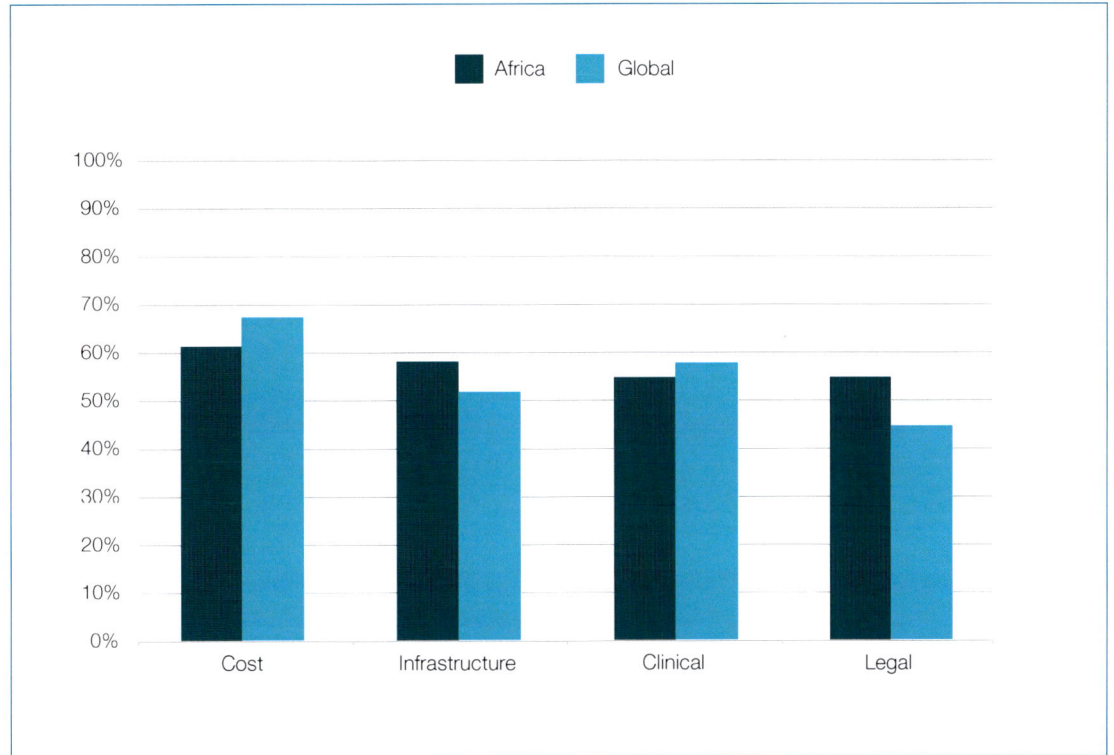

Figure 35. Information needs of the Eastern Mediterranean Region

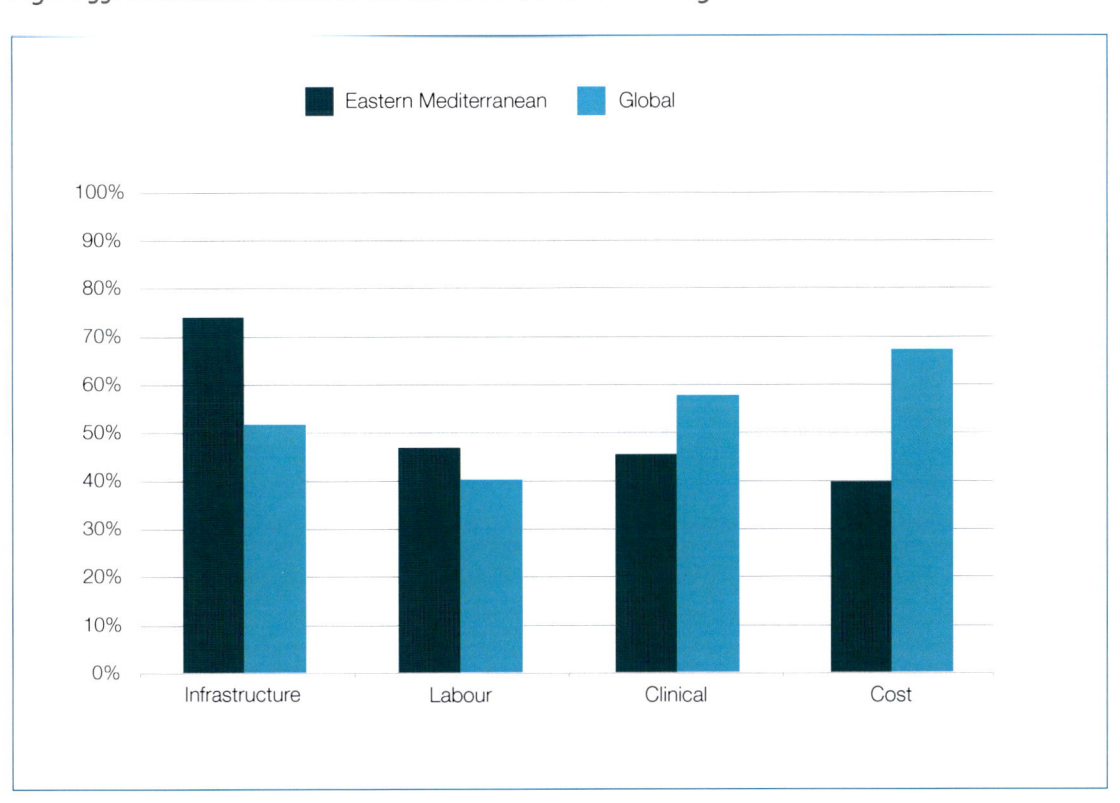

Figure 36. Information needs of the European Region

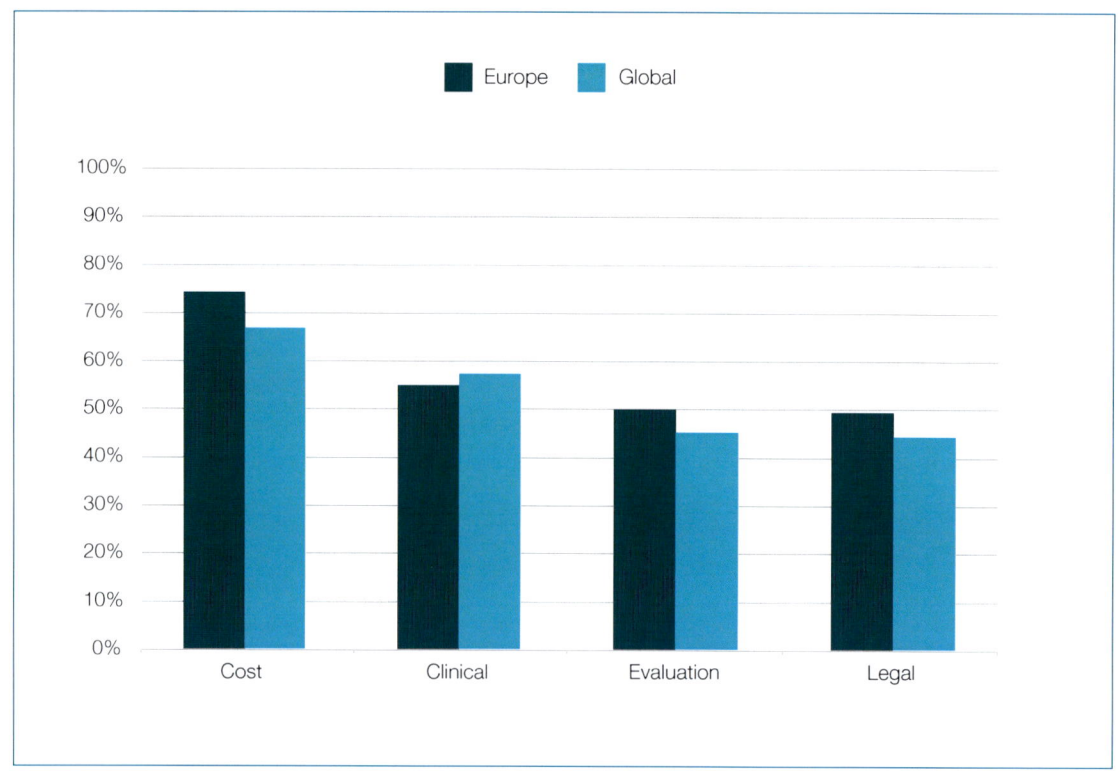

Figure 37. Information needs of the Region of the Americas

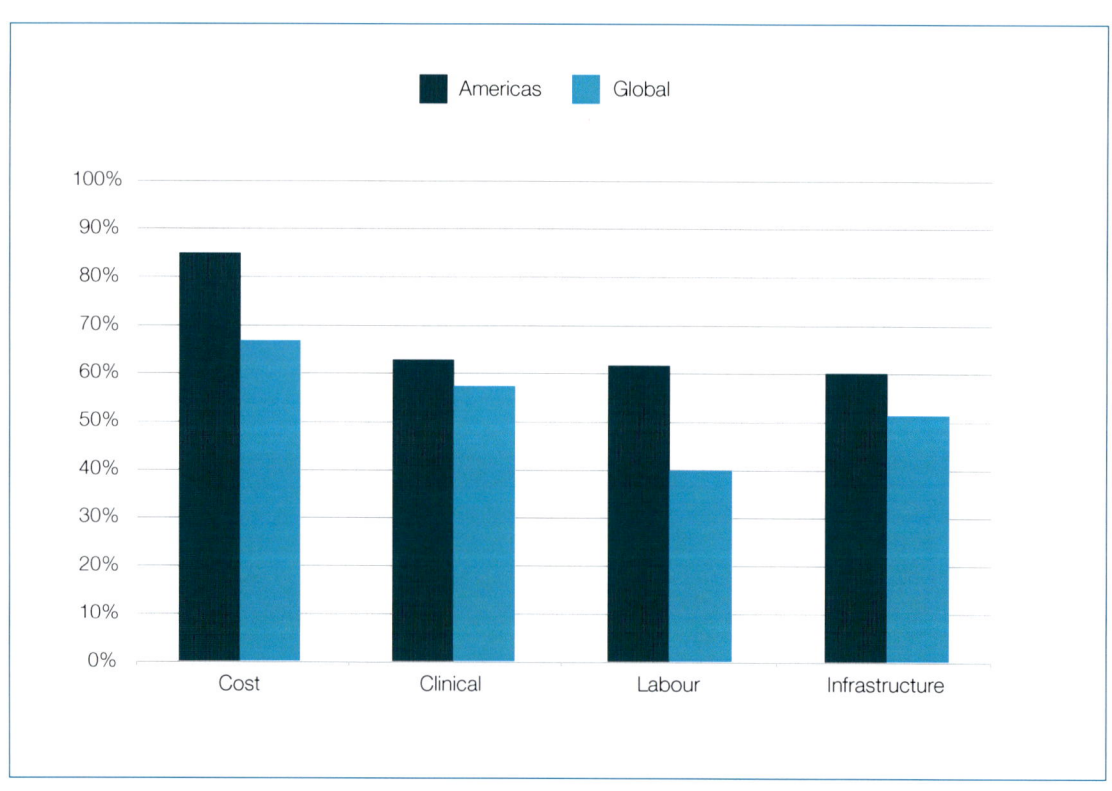

Figure 38. Information needs of the South-East Asia Region

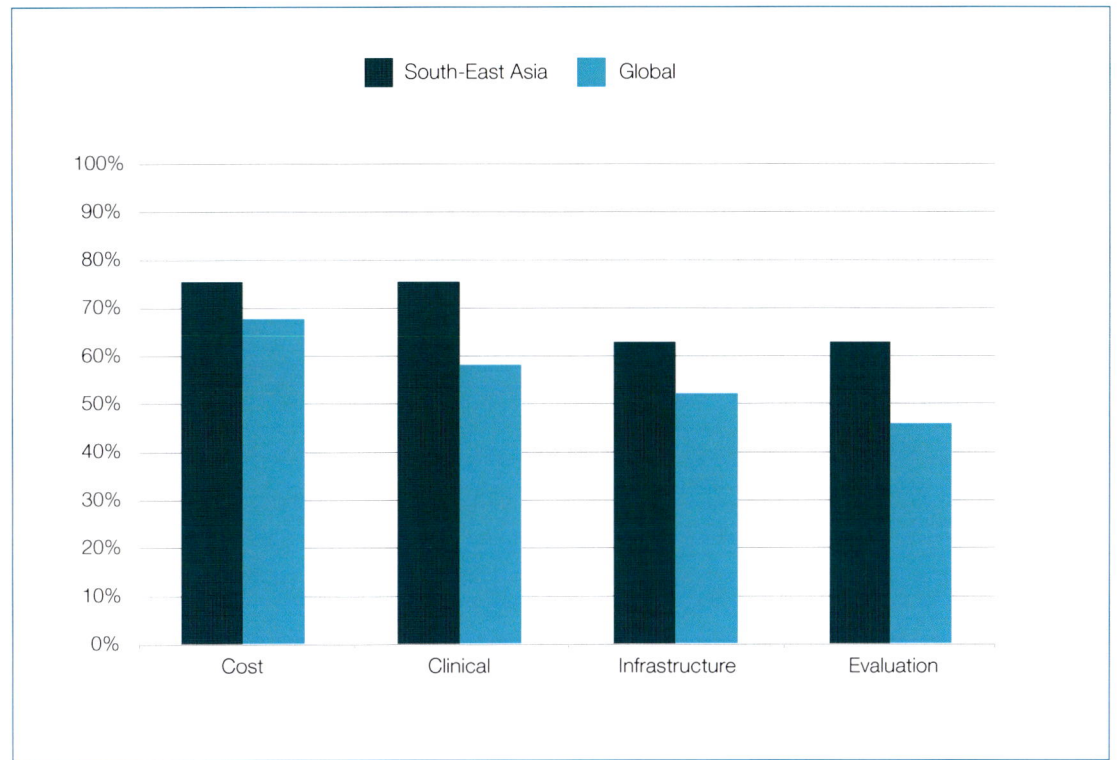

Figure 39. Information needs of the Western Pacific Region

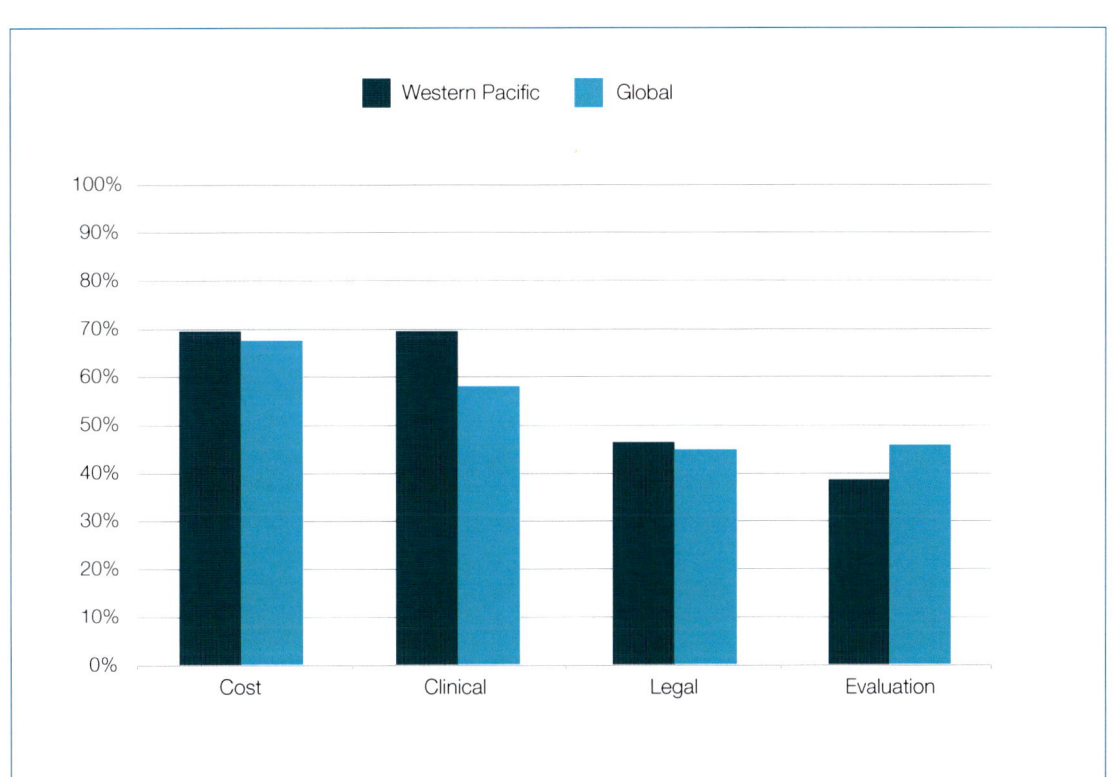

Figure 40 shows the information needs for telemedicine classified by World Bank income group. All seven options from the survey have been presented together to better illustrate trends between information needs and country income levels.

Results by income group were similar to the trends found by WHO region. With regards to cost and resource issues, it is of interest to note that the proportion of countries requiring more information on cost and cost-effectiveness of telemedicine ranged between 60% and 75%, with the highest proportion reported by high-income countries. Naturally, infrastructure appears to be a greater issue among low-income countries than those in the high-income group, 70% and 35%, respectively.

Cost and infrastructure were the most commonly cited information needs by low-income countries, while less than 20% reported information on patients' perception of, or satisfaction with, telemedicine as being an important information need. High-income countries appeared less likely to need information on the legal and ethical aspects of telemedicine, a finding worthy of note when one considers that developed countries often considered legal issues surrounding patient privacy and confidentiality to be a barrier to telemedicine implementation. The relatively high interest in information on the clinical possibilities for the use of telemedicine appears largely driven by countries in the upper-middle income group; almost 80% of countries in this group required more information on this area, about 25% higher than any other income group.

Figure 40. Information needs by World Bank income group

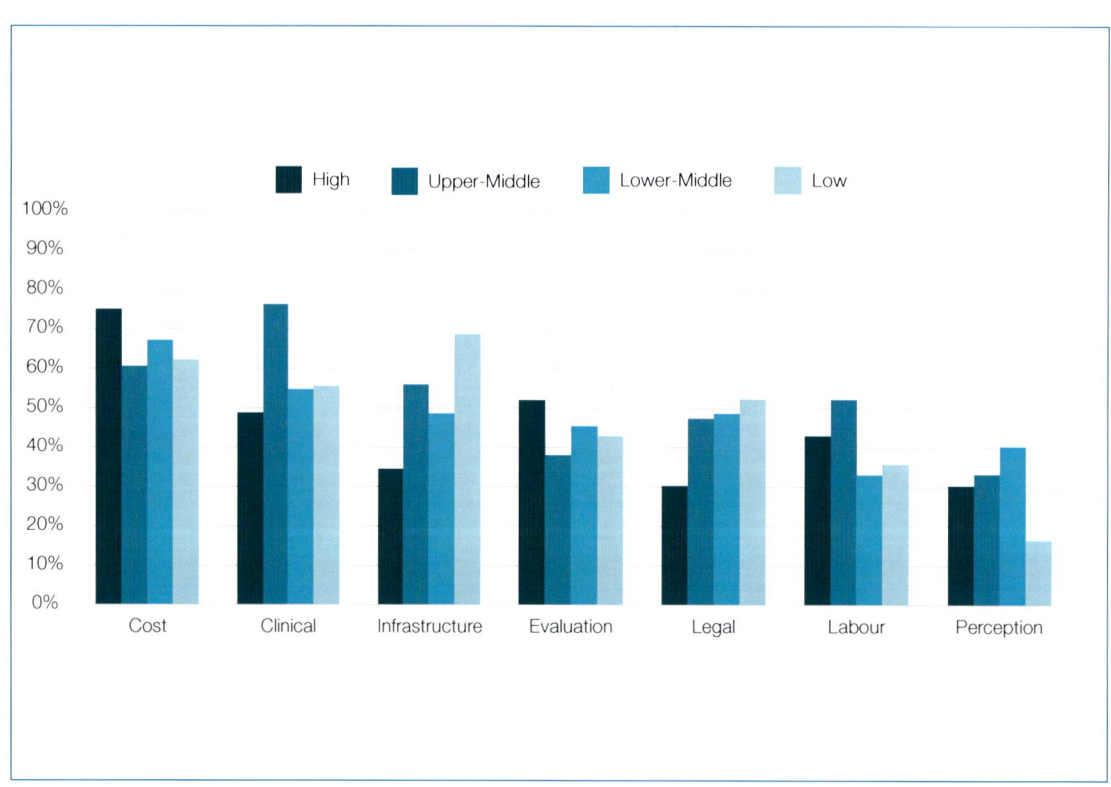

### 4.4.1 Implications for the information needs of telemedicine

Generally speaking, similar kinds of information needs are present irrespective of a country's current income or level of telemedicine uptake. It is possible that the information needs of a country depend more on their particular health care system requirements, and less on the economic resources available to them. While in most regions addressing economic and resource concerns appear to be a priority, there is also a clear need to provide information and education at the global level on the breadth of medical specialties where telemedicine solutions are viable. The results suggest that more documentation of evidence of telemedicine, best practices, cost-effectiveness analysis, and health policies to govern and stimulate demand for telemedicine services would fill the needs of countries in all regions and all income levels.

The request for more information regarding the costs and cost-effectiveness of telemedicine solutions from high-income countries, and the high demand for more information on the clinical use of telemedicine by upper-middle-income countries exemplify these specific needs. A potential explanation for this finding is that in developed countries, where access to health care services is not as critical an issue and consumers have a broader choice of services, greater scrutiny is placed on other aspects of telemedicine services to justify its adoption. These aspects may include its potential cost-effectiveness, clinical utility, and its effect on human resources in health care.

In developing countries, where access to health care services can be scarce, and where there is commonly a critical shortage of human resources for health and clinical services, increased access is a strong incentive for telemedicine implementation. However, this heightened need for good quality basic medical service diminishes the relative need for information on areas such as cost-effectiveness. This is further illustrated by the very low proportion of low-income countries that wanted more information on patients' perception of telemedicine. In these countries, the provision of, and access to services has far greater priority over how the service recipients perceive them. The results also reflect the fact that the infrastructure required to implement telemedicine is of vital importance to developing countries, and that this is an area of needed information and support. To this end, additional high-quality evaluations and studies should be conducted to build the evidence base for the best use of available resources, especially when those resources are scarce.

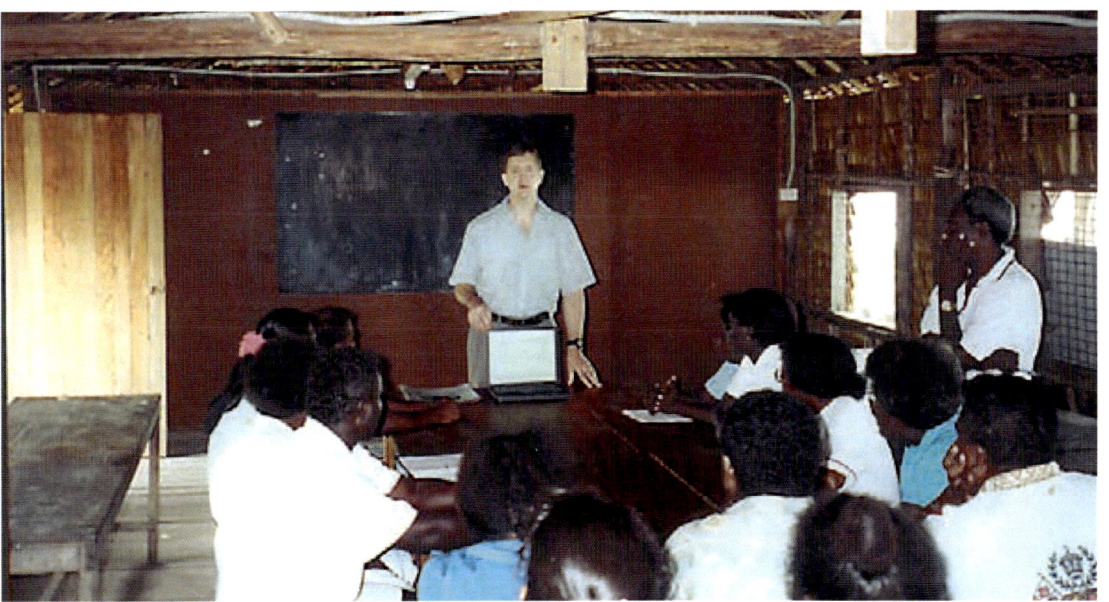

*Teaching principles of eHealth to nursing staff at the Gizo Hospital in the Solomon Islands. (Photograph: Swinfen Charitable Trust)*

# 5. Discussion and recommendations

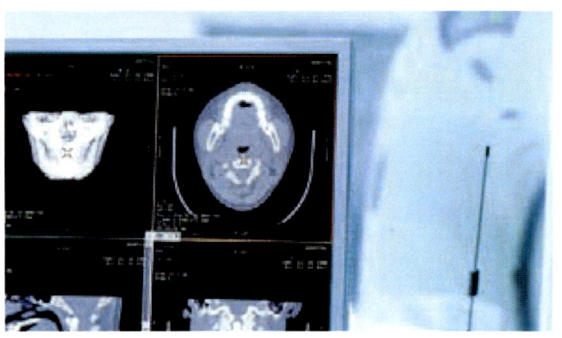
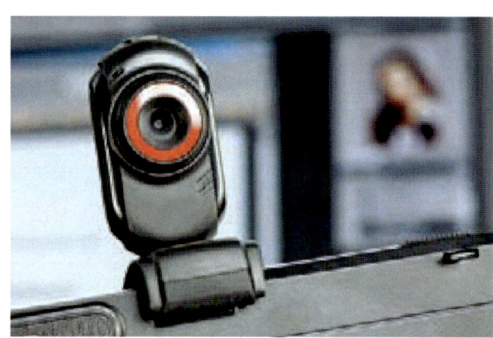
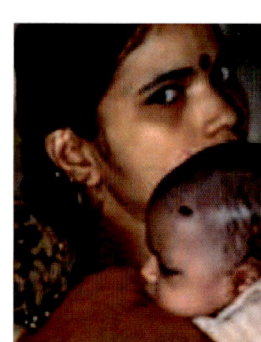

## 5.1 The current state of telemedicine services

Overall, the findings of this survey indicate that provision of telemedicine is far less progressed in upper-middle, lower-middle and low-income countries than in high-income countries, with respect to both the proportion of countries with established services and the proportion of countries offering telemedicine services. Of the four fields of telemedicine that were highlighted in the survey (teleradiology, telepathology, teledermatology, and telepsychiatry), teleradiology – a relatively simple store-and-forward telemedicine solution – has the highest rate of established service provision.

The survey examined the status of a number of factors facilitating telemedicine development as well as barriers to telemedicine development. The following recommendations address the findings of these key factors.

### 5.1.1 Factors facilitating telemedicine development

Effective agencies could be used to help define the vision and objectives of national telemedicine policies and direct efforts towards implementation within countries. Yet only 30% of responding countries reported having a national agency for the development and promotion of telemedicine, and 20% reported having developed and implemented a national telemedicine policy. These results suggest the need for Member States to prioritize the establishment of a national telemedicine governing body or agency to guide a strategy for the development, implementation, and evaluation of telemedicine solutions.

Such work would best be accomplished through collaboration between all stakeholders—policymakers, health administrators, health professionals, academic institutions, and communities. This could affirm the place of telemedicine in the current health system, and identify the gaps in health care that telemedicine can address. Teams working within a region or community would be best positioned to understand specific regional or national clinical approaches, legal frameworks, and cultural approaches to health services delivery. In addition to identifying community strengths and resilience in solving gaps in care through telemedicine solutions, these teams would also be instrumental in informing future telemedicine development and evolution. Collaboration includes international institutions so that innovative ideas and practices brought from outside the local context could be introduced and integrated with local support.

Collaboration also applies to the scientific institutions involved with the development of telemedicine solutions. With these groups, particularly, and with all telemedicine generally, results show the need for rigorous evaluation to inform policy and strategy. Evaluation should be identified as a necessary and important component of any telemedicine project design, and the evaluation framework should be meaningful to all telemedicine stakeholders including decision-makers for telemedicine policy, health care administrators responsible for quality improvement, and health-care professionals responsible for providing evidence-based care.

Evaluations, however, do little unless they are published and their results acted upon. Effective dissemination of evaluation results and their integration into routine practice as part of the health system is critical to the success of telemedicine programmes. WHO defines such 'knowledge translation' as "the synthesis, exchange and application of knowledge by relevant stakeholders to accelerate the benefits of global and local innovation in strengthening health systems and improving people's health" (87). Effective knowledge translation using an equity-orientated framework to tailor relevant interventions to specific audiences could be a sound strategy in advancing telemedicine uptake (87).

Table 7 lists WHO's recommendations to facilitate the development of telemedicine in Member States. Based on the results of the 2009 eHealth Survey, these recommendations are presented alongside WHO actions to foster eHealth development worldwide.

Table 7. Recommendations to Member States to facilitate telemedicine development

| WHO actions | Recommendations to Member States |
|---|---|
| **Governance** | |
| The fifty-eighth World Health Assembly in May 2005 adopted resolution WHA58.28 establishing an eHealth strategy for WHO. | WHO urges Member States to consider long-term strategic plans for the development and implementation of eHealth services which include telemedicine. It calls on governments to form national eHealth bodies to provide guidance in policy and strategy, data security, legal and ethical issues, interoperability, cultural and linguistic issues, infrastructure, funding, as well as monitoring and evaluation.<br><br>WHO recommends that Member States establish a national-level body for eHealth, supported by the ministry of health, as an instrument for implementing the WHA eHealth resolution. The body should include a division responsible for the governance of telemedicine and advocating for services at the local level to address pressing health concerns. |
| **Policy and strategy** | |
| WHO and its partners will develop a set of tools and guidelines on a comprehensive eHealth policy that includes telemedicine, for adaptation and adoption by Member States. | WHO recommends that Member States adapt to local contexts eHealth policies that include the use of telemedicine. Member States are encouraged to inform policy by engaging stakeholders at all levels: community, health professionals, academic institutions, health administrators, and policy-makers. |
| **Scientific development and evaluation** | |
| To stimulate knowledge translation, WHO will work with stakeholders to develop a framework for evaluation including suitable indicators and will build a registry of selected research findings for telemedicine. This registry will provide an incentive for the scientific community to contribute to the telemedicine knowledge and evidence base. | WHO recommends that Member States support and encourage telemedicine research and evaluation initiatives that include methodologies and strategies for knowledge translation. Funded projects should incorporate an evaluation framework that is meaningful to all telemedicine stakeholders. |

## 5.1.2 Barriers to telemedicine development

The most frequently reported barrier to the implementation of telemedicine solutions was the perception that telemedicine programmes were too expensive to implement. While this is true for some programmes, others, as discussed above, can be implemented using pre-existing infrastructure and are therefore relatively inexpensive. For example, asynchronous store-and-forward measures such as e-mail services have been found to be usable in areas with limited bandwidth to successfully deliver telemedicine across a variety of medical specialties and international environments. Still, this finding emphasizes the need to build on existing resources and infrastructure, and introduce other simple, low-cost telemedicine solutions within the context of the community to provide the basis for evaluation and further adoption. Start-up costs should be kept as low as possible to increase the likelihood of committed funding to support new innovations. Table 8 illustrates actions WHO recommends to overcome these barriers.

Underdeveloped infrastructure was a common barrier to telemedicine development particularly cited by developing countries. To address this issue, infrastructure development should be planned to benefit societies in ways beyond health, such as e-government, e-commerce, or eLearning. For example, applications created for telemedicine services can be used for government-related meetings and planning or can be used to connect schools in the area to enhance educational experiences. Understanding how the electronic infrastructure adds to community resilience, and how telemedicine applications may not only be a beneficiary of electronic infrastructure, but also an active contributor to a growing list of electronic applications for community members, would be a highly important exercise to ensure long-term sustainability of telemedicine projects. WHO urges Member States to enable the development and use of innovative telemedicine solutions to assist health-care professionals working in both urban and rural areas to provide community-specific services, including mobile telemedicine solutions. Recommendations for the use of mobile eHealth technologies are discussed in the mHealth report, a part of the GOe eHealth series (forthcoming).

Finally, many developed countries reported concerns regarding legal issues such as those associated with ensuring patient confidentiality. For support in establishing legal policies, Member States are encouraged to refer to the legal report (forthcoming), which forms a part of the GOe eHealth series.

Table 8. Actions Member States can take to overcome barriers to telemedicine development

| Barriers to telemedicine development | |
|---|---|
| WHO actions | Recommendations to Member States |
| Cost and infrastructure | |
| WHO will collect and disseminate examples of economically viable telemedicine solutions, particularly for low-income settings, to facilitate the uptake of appropriate telemedicine solutions. | WHO recommends that Member States invest in cost-effective, multipurpose telemedicine solutions. To keep solutions feasible, telemedicine applications should be adapted to local ICT and infrastructure; these applications should be funded as part of an integrated health service delivery strategy. To maximize affordability and sustainability of infrastructure development, WHO recommends that Member States foster global, national, and regional collaboration and partnerships. This may include partnerships with private and nongovernmental sectors with the protection of legally binding agreements. |
| Information needs | |
| WHO and partners will facilitate the flow of information by supporting forums on telemedicine to inform policy-makers and users of telemedicine programmes. The GOe will continue to disseminate strategic information to Member States on telemedicine applications, best practice, and evaluation. | WHO recommends that Member States convene a forum with ministries of health, the ICT sector, education and other stakeholders to discuss how telemedicine can improve health care delivery. Member States are encouraged to include ICT training of health-care professionals in curricula, to familiarize them with telemedicine solutions. |

# References

1. Strehle EM, Shabde N. One hundred years of telemedicine: does this new technology have a place in paediatrics? *Archives of Disease in Childhood*, 2006, 91(12):956–959.

2. Sood SP, et al. Differences in public and private sector adoption of telemedicine: Indian case study for sectoral adoption. *Studies in Health Technology and Informatics*, 2007, 130:257–268.

3. WHO. *A health telematics policy in support of WHO's Health-For-All strategy for global health development: report of the WHO group consultation on health telematics, 11–16 December, Geneva, 1997*. Geneva, World Health Organization, 1998.

4. Craig J, Patterson V. Introduction to the practice of telemedicine. *Journal of Telemedicine and Telecare*, 2005, 11(1):3–9.

5. Einthoven W. Le télécardiogramme [The telecardiogram]. *Archives Internationales de Physiologie*, 1906, 4:132–164.

6. Currell R et al. Telemedicine versus face to face patient care: effects on professional practice and health care outcomes. *Cochrane Database of Systematic Reviews*, 2000, Issue 2. Art. No.: CD002098.

7. Benschoter RA, Eaton MT, Smith P. Use of videotape to provide individual instruction in techniques of psychotherapy. *Academic Medicine*, 1965, 40(12):1159–1161.

8. Dwyer TF. Telepsychiatry: psychiatric consultation by interactive television. *American Journal of Psychiatry*, 1973, 130:865–869.

9. Wootton R, Jebamani LS, Dow SA. E-health and the Universitas 21 organization: 2. Telemedicine and underserved populations. *Journal of Telemedicine and Telecare*, 2005, 11(5):221–224.

10. Rao B, Lombardi A II. Telemedicine: current status in developed and developing countries. *Journal of Drugs in Dermatology*, 2009, 8(4):371–375.

11. Wootton R, Menzies J, Ferguson P. Follow-up data for patients managed by store and forward telemedicine in developing countries. *Journal of Telemedicine and Telecare*, 2009, 15(2):83–88.

12. Wootton R. The development of telemedicine. In: Rigby, Roberts, Thick, eds. *Taking Health Telematics into the 21st Century*. Oxon, Radcliffe Medical Press, 2000:17–26.

13. Heinzelmann PJ, Lugn NE, Kvedar JC. Telemedicine in the future. *Journal of Telemedicine and Telecare*, 2005, 11(8):384–390.

14. Wootton R. Telemedicine support for the developing world. *Journal of Telemedicine and Telecare*, 2008, 14(3):109–114.

15. Jennett PA et al. The socio-economic impact of telehealth: a systematic review. *Journal of Telemedicine and Telecare*, 2003, 9(6):311–320.

16. al Shorbaji N. e-Health in the Eastern Mediterranean region: A decade of challenges and achievements. *East Mediterranean Health Journal*, 2008, 14(Supp.):S157–S173.

17. Kifle M, Mbarika V, Datta P. Telemedicine in sub-Saharan Africa: The case of teleophthalmology and eye care in Ethiopia. *Journal of the American Society for Information Science & Technology*, 2006, 57(10):1383–1393.

18. Swanepoel D, Olusanya B, Mars M. Hearing health-care delivery in sub-Saharan Africa – a role for tele-audiology. *Journal of Telemedicine and Telecare*, 2010, 16(2):53–56.

19. Swinfen R, Swinfen P. Low-cost telemedicine in the developing world. *Journal of Telemedicine and Telecare*, 2002, 8(Suppl. 3):S63–65.
20. Qaddoumi I, Bouffet E. Supplementation of a successful pediatric neuro-oncology telemedicine-based twinning program by e-mails. *Telemedicine Journal and e-Health*, 2009, 15(10):975–982.
21. Stanberry B. Legal and ethical aspects of telemedicine. *Journal of Telemedicine and Telecare*, 2006, 12(4):166–175.
22. Resolution WHA58.28. eHealth. In: Fifty-eighth World Health Assembly, Geneva, May 16–25, 2005 (http://apps.who.int/gb/ebwha/pdf_files/WHA58/WHA58_28-en.pdf, accessed 17 June 2010).
23. Brandling-Bennett HA et al. Delivering health care in rural Cambodia via store-and-forward telemedicine: a pilot study. *Telemedicine Journal and e-Health*, 2005, 11(1):56–62.
24. Pradhan MR. ICTs application for better health in Nepal. *Kathmandu University Medical Journal*, 2004, 2(2):157–163.
25. Mishra A. Telemedicine in otolaryngology (an Indian perspective). *Indian Journal of Otolaryngology and Head and Neck Surgery*, 2003, 55(3):211–212.
26. Froelich W et al. 2009. Case report: an example of international telemedicine success. *Journal of Telemedicine and Telecare*, 2009, 15(4):208-210.
27. Vinals F et al. Prenatal diagnosis of congenital heart disease using four-dimensional spatio-temporal image correlation (STIC) telemedicine via an internet link: a pilot study. *Ultrasound in Obstetrics & Gynecology*, 2005, 25(1):25–31.
28. Kvedar J, Heinzelmann PJ, Jacques G. Cancer diagnosis and telemedicine: a case study from Cambodia. *Annals of Oncology*, 2006, 17(Suppl. 8):S37–S42.
29. Chanussot-Deprez C, Contreras-Ruiz J. Telemedicine in wound care. *International Wound Journal*, 2008, 5(5):651–654.
30. Benzion I, Helveston EM. Use of telemedicine to assist ophthalmologists in developing countries for the diagnosis and management of four categories of ophthalmic pathology. *Clinical Ophthalmology*, 2007, 1(4):489–495.
31. Mukundan S II et al. Trial telemedicine system for supporting medical students on elective in the developing world. *Academic Radiology*, 2003, 10(7):794–797.
32. Heinzelmann PJ, Jacques G, Kvedar JC. Telemedicine by email in remote Cambodia. *Journal of Telemedicine and Telecare*, 2005, 11(Suppl. 2):S44–S47.
33. Latifi R et al. «Initiate-build-operate-transfer» – a strategy for establishing sustainable telemedicine programs in developing countries: initial lessons from the Balkans. *Telemedicine and e-Health*, 2009, 15(14):956.
34. Vassallo DJ et al. An evaluation of the first year's experience with a low-cost telemedicine link in Bangladesh. *Journal of Telemedicine and Telecare*, 2001, 7(3):125–138.
35. Vassallo DJ et al. Experience with a low-cost telemedicine system in three developing countries. *Journal of Telemedicine and Telecare*, 2001, 7(Suppl. 1):S56–S58.
36. Gagnon MP et al. Implementing telehealth to support medical practice in rural/remote regions: What are the conditions for success? *Implementation Science*, 2006, 1:18.
37. Nakajima I, Chida S. Telehealth in the Pacific: current status and analysis report (1999-2000). *Journal of Medical Systems*, 2000, 24(6):321–331.
38. Geissbuhler A et al. Telemedicine in western Africa: Lessons learned from a pilot project in Mali: perspectives and recommendations. *AMIA Annual Symposium Proceedings*, 2003:249–253.
39. Martinez A et al. Analysis of information and communication needs in rural primary health care in developing countries. *IEEE Transactions on Information Technology in Biomedicine*, 2005, 9(1):66–72.
40. Zbar RI et al. Web-based medicine as a means to establish centers of surgical excellence in the developing world. *Plastic and Reconstructive Surgery*, 2001, 108(2):460–465.
41. Wootton R. Telemedicine and developing countries – successful implementation will require a shared approach. *Journal of Telemedicine and Telecare*, 2001, 7(Suppl. 1):S1–S6.
42. Qaddoumi I et al. Team management, twinning, and telemedicine in retinoblastoma: A 3-tier approach implemented in the first eye salvage program in Jordan. *Pediatric Blood & Cancer*, 2008, 51(2):241–244.
43. Bush LA et al. Adrenal insufficiency secondary to tuberculosis: The value of telemedicine in the remote diagnosis of Addison's disease in Ebeye, republic of the Marshall Islands. *Hawaii Medical Journal*, 2009, 68(1):8–11.
44. Brauchli K et al. iPath: a telemedicine platform to support health providers in low resource settings. *Journal on Information Technology in Healthcare*, 2005, 3(4):227–235.

45. Patterson V et al. Supporting hospital doctors in the Middle East by email telemedicine: something the industrialized world can do to help. *Journal of Medical Internet Research*, 2007, 9(4):e30.

46. Johnston K et al. The cost-effectiveness of technology transfer using telemedicine. *Health Policy and Planning*, 2004, 19(5):302–309.

47. Sozen C, Kisa A, Kavuncubasi S. Can rural telemedicine help to solve the health care access problems in Turkey? *Clinical Research and Regulatory Affairs*, 2003, 20(1):117–126.

48. Wootton R. Design and implementation of an automatic message-routing system for low-cost telemedicine. *Journal of Telemedicine and Telecare*, 2003, 9(Suppl. 1):S44–S47.

49. Swinfen P et al. A review of the first year's experience with an automatic message-routing system for low-cost telemedicine. *Journal of Telemedicine and Telecare*, 2003, 9(Suppl. 2):S63–S65.

50. Martinez A et al. A study of a rural telemedicine system in the Amazon region of Peru. *Journal of Telemedicine and Telecare*, 2004, 10(4):219–225.

51. Alverson DC et al. Transforming systems of care for children in the global community. *Pediatric Annal*, 2009, 38(10):579–585.

52. Seiwerth S, Danilovic Z. The telepathology and teleradiology network in Croatia. *Analytical Cellular Pathology*, 2000, 21(3–4):223–228.

53. Kiviat AD et al. HIV online provider education (HOPE): the Internet as a tool for training in HIV medicine. *The Journal of Infectious Diseases*, 2007, 196(Suppl. 3):S512–S515.

54. Lee S et al. The role of low-bandwidth telemedicine in surgical prescreening. *Journal of Pediatric Surgery*, 2003, 38(9):1281–1283.

55. Lanre AO, Makanjuola AT. Knowledge and perception of e-health and telemedicine among health professionals in LAUTECH teaching hospital, Osogbo, Nigeria. *International Journal of Health Research*, 2009, 2(1):51–58.

56. Khazei A et al. An assessment of the telehealth needs and health-care priorities of Tanna island: a remote, under-served and vulnerable population. *Journal of Telemedicine and Telecare*, 2005, 11(1):35–40.

57. Bagchi S. Telemedicine in rural India. *PLoS Medicine*, 2006, 3(3):e82.

58. Doarn CR, Adilova F, Lam D. A review of telemedicine in Uzbekistan. *Journal of Telemedicine and Telecare*, 2005, 11(3):135–139.

59. Durrani H, Khoja S. A systematic review of the use of telehealth in Asian countries. *Journal of Telemedicine and Telecare*, 2009, 15(4):175–181.

60. Stutchfield BM, Jagilly R, Tulloh BR. Second opinions in remote surgical practice using email and digital photography. *ANZ Journal of Surgery*, 2007, 77(11):1009–1012.

61. Zhao Y, Nakajima I, Juzoji H. On-site investigation of the early phase of Bhutan health telematics project. *Journal of Medical Systems*, 2002, 26(1): 67–77.

62. Pal A et al. Telemedicine diffusion in a developing country: the case of India. *IEEE Transactions on Information Technology in Biomedicine*, 2005, 9(1):59–65.

63. Xue Y, Liang H. Analysis of telemedicine diffusion: the case of China. *IEEE Transactions on Information Technology in Biomedicine*, 2007, 11(2):231–233.

64. Kaplan WA. Can the ubiquitous power of mobile phones be used to improve health outcomes in developing countries? *Globalization and Health*, 2006, 23(2):9.

65. Sood SP, Bhatia JS. Development of telemedicine technology in India: "Sanjeevani" – an integrated telemedicine application. *Journal of Postgraduate Medicine*, 2005, 51(4):308–311.

66. Abbas MI, Person DA. The Pacific Island health care project (PIHCP): experience with rheumatic heart disease (RHD) from 1998 to 2006. *Hawaii Medical Journal*, 2008, 67(12):326–329.

67. Thara R, John S, Rao K. Telepsychiatry in Chennai, India: The SCARF experience. *Behavioral Sciences & the Law*, 2008, 26(3):315–322.

68. Tomasi E, Facchini LA, Maia MF. Health information technology in primary health care in developing countries: a literature review. *Bulletin of the World Health Organization*, 2004, 82(11):867–874.

69. Pattynama PM. Legal aspects of cross-border teleradiology. *European Journal of Radiology*, 2010, 73(1):26–30.

70. Blaya JA, Fraser HS, Holt B. E-health technologies show promise in developing countries. *Health Affairs*, 2010, 29(2):244–251.

71. Tierney WM et al. A toolkit for e-health partnerships in low-income nations. *Health Affairs*, 2010, 29(2):268–273.

72. Geissbuhler A, Bagayoko CO, Ly O. The RAFT network: 5 years of distance continuing medical education and tele-consultations over the internet in French-speaking Africa. *International Journal of Medical Informatics*, 2007, 76(5-6):351–356.

73. el Gatit AM et al. Effects of an awareness symposium on perception of Libyan physicians regarding telemedicine. *East Mediterranean Health Journal*, 2008, 14(4):926–930.

74. Mireskandari M et al. Teleconsultation in diagnostic pathology: experience from Iran and Germany with the use of two European telepathology servers. Journal of Telemedicine and Telecare, 2004, 10(2):99–103.

75. Person DA, Hedson JS, Gunawardane KJ. Telemedicine success in the United States Associated Pacific Islands (USAPI): Two illustrative cases. *Telemedicine Journal and e-Health*, 2003, 9(1):95–101.

76. Szot A et al. Diagnostic accuracy of chest X-rays acquired using a digital camera for low-cost teleradiology. *International Journal of Medical Informatics*, 2004, 73(1):65–73.

77. Patterson V et al. Store-and-forward teleneurology in developing countries. *Journal of Telemedicine and Telecare*, 2001, 7(Suppl. 1):S52–S53.

78. Qaddoumi I et al. Impact of telemedicine on pediatric neuro-oncology in a developing country: the Jordanian-Canadian experience. *Pediatric Blood & Cancer*, 2007, 48(1):39–43.

79. Pradeep PV et al. Reinforcement of endocrine surgery training: impact of telemedicine technology in a developing country context. *World Journal of Surgery*, 2007, 31(8):1665–1671.

80. Sørensen T, Rivett U, Fortuin J. A review of ICT systems for HIV/AIDS and anti-retroviral treatment management in South Africa. *Journal of Telemedicine and Telecare*, 2008, 14(1):37–41.

81. First Nations Centre. OCAP: *Ownership, Control, Access, and Possession.* Sanctioned by the First Nations Information Governance Committee, Assembly of First Nations. Ottawa, National Aboriginal Health Organization, 2007 (http://www.naho.ca/firstnations/english/documents/toolkits/FNC_OCAPInformationResource.pdf, accessed 30 June 2010).

82. Berwick DM, Nolan TW, Whittington J. The triple aim: care, health, and cost. *Health Affairs*, 2008, 27(3):759–769.

83. Gerber T et al. An agenda for action on global e-health. *Health Affairs*, 2010, 29(2):233–236.

84. Wootton R et al. Prospective case review of a global e-health system for doctors in developing countries. *Journal of Telemedicine and Telecare*, 2004, 10(Suppl. 1):S94–S96.

85. Misra UK et al. Telemedicine in neurology: underutilized potential. *Neurology India*, 2005, 53(1):27–31.

86. Zolfo M et al. Remote consultations and HIV/AIDS continuing education in low-resource settings. *International Journal of Medical Informatics*, 2006, 75(9):633–637.

87. WHO. *Bridging the "know–do" gap: meeting on knowledge translation in global health.* Geneva, World Health Organization, 2006 (WHO/EIP/KMS/2006.2; http://www.who.int/kms/WHO_EIP_KMS_2006_2.pdf, accessed 12 July 2010).

# Appendix 1

Country-reported services provided through telemedicine

| Country | Institutions / Service providers | Stage |
|---|---|---|
| **Biochemistry** | | |
| Turkey | Information Technologies Department | Established |
| **Cardiology / Electrocardiography** | | |
| Austria | Medical University of Graz | Pilot |
| | Austrian Institute of Technology GmbH | Pilot |
| | Austrian Research Centers GmbH | Pilot |
| Belarus | Республиканский научно-практический центр «»Кардиология»» | Established |
| Belgium | Saint John Hospital, Brussels | Established |
| Bhutan | Jigme Dorji Wangchuck National Referral Hospital | Established |
| Burundi | Le Centre Hospitalo – Universitaire de Kamenge | Pilot |
| Cape Verde | Hospital Pediatrico de Coimbra, Servico de Cardiologia Pediatrica | Established |
| Colombia | Fundación Cardiovascular de Colombia | Established |
| Croatia | Institute of Telemedicine | Established |
| Czech Republic | Institut Klinické a Experimentální Medicíny | Pilot |
| Estonia | Tartu University Hospital | Established |
| Greece | Biomedical Research Foundation of the Academy of Athens, Biotechnology Division, Bioinformatics & Medical Informatics Team | Pilot |
| Iceland | Landspitali University Hospital | Pilot |
| Indonesia | National Cardiovascular Center Harapan Kita | Established |
| Latvia | Telemedica | Informal |

| Country | Institutions / Service providers | Stage |
|---|---|---|
| Malaysia | Ministry of Health, Telehealth Division | Pilot |
| Mali | Agence National de Telemedicine et Informatique Medical | — |
| Mexico | Serviciois Estatales de Salud y Universidades | Established |
| Mongolia | Shastin Central Hospital | Established |
| Mozambique | Hospital Central de Maputo e Beira | Pilot |
| Nepal | Patan Hospital | Established |
| Norway | Norwegian Centre for Integrated Care and Telemedicine | Established |
| New Zealand | Vivid Solutions | Established |
| Pakistan | Holy Family Hospital, Rawalpindi | Established |
| Paraguay | Instituto de Investigaciones en Ciencias de la Salud – Universidad Nacional de Asunción | Pilot |
| Peru | ITMS Perú (Telemedicina de Perú S.A.) | Established |
| Peru | Instituto Nacional de Investigación y Capacitación de Telecomunicaciones – Ministerio de Salud | Pilot |
| Senegal | Fann Hospital | Established |
| Singapore | Singapore General Hospital, Accident and Emergency Department | Pilot |
| Turkey | Information Technologies Department | Established |
| **Consultation** | | |
| France | Centre Hospitalier de Versailles / Etablissement Pénitentiaire de Bois d'Arcy | Established |
| Nepal | Patan Hospital | Established |
| New Zealand | Vivid Solutions | Established |
| Niger | Hopital Régional de Tahoua | Pilot |
| Niger | Hopital de District de Mainé Soroa | Pilot |
| Nigeria | Herzliya Medical Center VI | — |
| Norway | Norwegian Centre for Integrated Care and Telemedicine | Established |
| Panama | Ministerio de Salud | Established |
| **Cytology** | | |
| Cyprus | Nicosia General Hospital | Established |
| **Dentistry** | | |
| Burkina Faso | Not reported | Established |
| **Diabetes** | | |
| Congo | Diabaction-Congo | Pilot |
| Germany | PHTS Telemedizin | Established |
| Germany | BKK Taunus | Established |

| Country | Institutions / Service providers | Stage |
|---|---|---|
| Mali | Agence National de Telemedicine et Informatique Medical | Informal |
| Greece | Sismanoglio General Hospital of Attica, Telemedicine Unit | Established |
| **Emergency medicine** | | |
| Croatia | Institute of Telemedicine | Pilot |
| **Haematology** | | |
| Czech Republic | Masaryk University, Faculty of Medicine | Established |
| **Hepatology** | | |
| Greece | Sismanoglio General Hospital of Attica, Telemedicine Unit | Established |
| **Histopathology** | | |
| Cyprus | Nicosia General Hospital | Established |
| **Home care** | | |
| Canada | Ontario Telemedicine Network, Province of Ontario | Pilot |
| Switzerland | Canton of Basel | Pilot |
| United Kingdom | Department of Health (with Kent, Newham, Cornwall) | Pilot |
| United Kingdom | National Health Service, Croydon | Established |
| United Kingdom | Cornwall Adult Social Care | Established |
| **Immunology** | | |
| New Zealand | Vivid Solutions | Established |
| **Laboratory services** | | |
| Switzerland | Canton of Ticino | Pilot |
| **Mammography** | | |
| Albania | Poliambulatorio Istituto Dermatologico dell'Immacolata, Tirana | Pilot |
| Austria | Tyrolean Telemedicine Project | Pilot |
| Belgium | IRIS Hospital Network | Established |
| Botswana | Botswana Government | Pilot |
| Burundi | Le Centre Hospitalo – Universitaire de Kamenge | Pilot |
| Country | Institutions / Service providers | Stage |
| Canada | Province of New Brunswick | Established |
| Estonia | Mammograaf Ltd. | Established |
| Germany | Klinikum Aschaffenburg | Established |
| India | Sir Ganga Ram Hospital | Established |
| Mexico | Servicios Estatales de Salud y Universidades | Established |
| New Zealand | Vivid Solutions | Established |
| Norway | Norwegian Centre for Integrated Care and Telemedicine | Established |

| Country | Institutions / Service providers | Stage |
|---|---|---|
| **Patient monitoring** | | |
| Canada | Saint John Regional Hospital, New Brunswick | Pilot |
| Colombia | Universidad Nacional de Colombia | — |
| Iceland | Landspitali University Hospital | Pilot |
| Uzbekistan | Ташкентский институт усовершенствования врачей | Pilot |
| **Nephrology** | | |
| Cameroon | Centre Hospitalier Universitaire de Yaoundé | Established |
| Canada | Province of New Brunswick | Established |
| Croatia | Institute of Telemedicine | Pilot |
| France | Centre Hospitalier Universitaire de Nancy | Established |
| Norway | Norwegian Centre for Integrated Care and Telemedicine | Established |
| **Neurology** | | |
| Croatia | Institute of Telemedicine | Pilot |
| Germany | HELIOS Hospital Group | Pilot |
| Senegal | Fann Hospital | Established |
| **Neurosurgery** | | |
| Czech Republic | Masaryk University, Faculty of Medicine | Established |
| Malaysia | Ministry of Health, Telehealth Division | Pilot |
| Pakistan | Jinnah Postgraduate Medical Center | — |
| **Obstetrics & gynaecology** | | |
| Bhutan | Jigme Dorji Wangchuck National Referral Hospital | Established |
| Bulgaria | Sheynovo Hospital, Sofia | Pilot |
| Burkina Faso | Not reported | Established |
| Iceland | Landspitali University Hospital | Pilot |
| Nepal | Patan Hospital | Established |
| **Oncology** | | |
| India | Regional Cancer Centre, Trivandrum | Established |
| Mali | Agence National de Telemedicine et Informatique Medical | — |
| **Ophthalmology** | | |
| Bhutan | Jigme Dorji Wangchuck National Referral Hospital | Established |
| Ethiopia | Federal Ministry of Health | Informal |
| France | Hôpital Lariboisière | Established |
| Indonesia | Cicendo Eye Hospital | Pilot |
| Mali | L'Institut d'Ophtalmologie Tropicale d'Afrique | Informal |

| Country | Institutions / Service providers | Stage |
|---|---|---|
| Philippines | University of the Philippines College of Medicine | Pilot |
| **Otolaryntology** | | |
| Burkina Faso | Not reported | Established |
| Pakistan | Holy Family Hospital, Rawalpindi | — |
| **Paediatrics** | | |
| Armenia | Arabkir Joint Medical Center | Established |
| Greece | Venizeleio-Pananio General Hospital | Established |
| Mongolia | Maternal and Child Health Research Center | Established |
| **Prostheses** | | |
| Philippines | National Telehealth Center | Pilot |
| Philippines | University of Philippines College of Medicine | Pilot |
| **Rehabilitation** | | |
| Slovenia | Institute for Rehabilitation | Pilot |
| **Rheumatology** | | |
| New Zealand | Vivid Solutions | Established |
| **Scintillography** | | |
| Paraguay | Instituto de Investigaciones en Ciencias de la Salud – Universidad Nacional de Asunción | Pilot |
| **Speech pathology** | | |
| Canada | Government of the Northwest Territories, Department of Health And Social Services | Pilot |
| **Stroke treatment** | | |
| Finland | Helsinki University Central Hospital | Established |
| Canada | Province of New Brunswick | Established |
| **Surgery** | | |
| Albania | University Hospital Mother Theresa, Tirana | Pilot |
| Bulgaria | Military Medical Academy | Informal |
| Bulgaria | UMBAL | Informal |
| Burkina Faso | Not reported | Established |
| Burundi | Le Centre Hospitalo – Universitaire de Kamenge | Pilot |
| France | Centre Hospitalier Universitaire de Strasbourg | Pilot |
| Greece | Hippokrateion Hospital, Athens | Pilot |
| India | Sanjay Gandhi Postgraduate Institute of Medical Sciences, School of Telemedicine & Biomedical Informatics | Established |
| Mali | Centre Hospitalier Universitaire Point-G, Service de Colio-Chirurgie | Pilot |

| Country | Institutions / Service providers | Stage |
|---|---|---|
| Norway | Norwegian Centre for Integrated Care and Telemedicine | Established |
| Pakistan | Holy Family Hospital, Rawalpindi | — |
| Turkmenistan | научно-исследовательский институт глазных болезней им.С.Каранова | Pilot |
| **Ultrasonography** | | |
| Afghanistan | Locknow Hospital | Established |
| Afghanistan | Chandighar Hospital | Established |
| Belarus | Государственное научное учреждение «Объединенный институт проблем информатики» Национальной академии наук Беларуси | Established |
| Botswana | Botswana Government | Pilot |
| Burkina Faso | Not reported | Established |
| Burundi | Le Centre Hospitalo – Universitaire de Kamenge | Pilot |
| France | Centre Hospitalier Universitaire de Grenoble | Established |
| Germany | Charité - Universitätsmedizin Berlin | Established |
| Iceland | Landspitali University Hospital | Established |
| Mexico | Serviciois Estatales de Salud y Universidades | Established |
| Nepal | Patan Hospital | Established |
| Pakistan | Holy Family Hospital, Rawalpindi | Established |
| Paraguay | Instituto de Investigaciones en Ciencias de la Salud – Universidad Nacional de Asunción | Pilot |
| Senegal | Fann Hospital | Established |
| Sudan | Not reported | Pilot |
| Turkey | Information Technologies Department | Pilot |
| **Urology** | | |
| Armenia | Yerevan State Medical University | Established |
| Greece | Sismanoglio General Hospital of Attica, Telemedicine Unit | Established |